FOLLOW ME

Follow Me
Anthony's Ultimate Journey

Ken Allbon

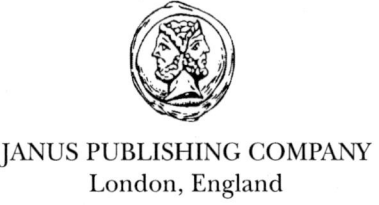

JANUS PUBLISHING COMPANY
London, England

First published in Great Britain 2009
by Janus Publishing Company Ltd,
105–107 Gloucester Place,
London W1U 6BY

www.januspublishing.co.uk

British Library Cataloguing-in-Publication Data
A catalogue record for this book is available from the British Library

ISBN 978-1-85756-780-9

Cover Design: Ken Allbon

Printed and bound in Great Britain

Dedication

For Gill, Michael and Katie
with my love

Contents

Foreword

This book reads easily from the word go. And if we are intent on a ready-made excitement or on being carried into values above the everyday, then the book will challenge us. Both are there, but they will not be fathomed without a readiness to go deeper into ourselves than is perhaps our daily custom: a readiness to place our hand into Anthony's for a while.

There is apparent, in this boy, the mystery that goes with being human. Anthony seemed to carry this around with him to a marked degree. We sense this more than all else in Ken Allbon's account of Anthony's life. Meeting him when he was 12 or 13 years old was to meet with an easiness of manner that was contagious, with a sense of humour that betokened life; life, which as we go through Anthony's remaining two years, was always beyond anything that death could threaten.

Anthony's school friends sensed something in him that they wanted. Perhaps this, more than anything else, was a willingness to give of himself.

We thank God for Anthony's life and death; for his death, because it is through his dying that we are most aware of his life. We are brought full circle to this Christian paradox, through a delightful 15-year-old schoolboy, who is now with God.

Brother George Linnegar,
Priest of St. Thomas a Becket Church, Cliffe, Lewes, July 2008

Acknowledgements

How the manuscript for this book actually came to be written down, I cannot say with any clarity. It started as a brief and inadequate list of possible chapter headings, immediately set aside and remaining untouched for many months. When I returned to the task, it was as one called by an irresistible voice; the words came with some rapidity and I wrote them down rather too quickly. Thus, the inspiration was from elsewhere and the inadequacies are entirely my own. Fortunately, in preparing the text for publication, I have been helped by many others to whom I owe a great debt of gratitude.

My special thanks go to four people who knew and loved Anthony. Without their encouragement, skills and dedication, my account of his journey would have been neither complete nor completed. Anthony will be joyous that these people, whom he valued so highly, have made a contribution to his story. Knowing me so well, he will appreciate, with a twinkle in his eye, how essential has been the gift of their work:

- Br George Linnegar for writing the Foreword and for his constant prayers, kindness, advice and, not least, his confident and frequent enquiries about when he was going to see the book. His clear perception of the significance of Anthony's witness has been of fundamental support in its writing.

- John Boyden, who has proofread the text with much patience and made many helpful suggestions. I am delighted that John, Anthony's English master, should have made such a contribution to this book about him.

- Mary Chandler, my typing and word-processing expert. Without Mary's tenacity and skill, and her valuable advice on textual improvement, the manuscript would not have been brought to a presentable state.

- Br Francis Edwards, who nursed Anthony during the darkest days of his illness, for his encouragement and for referring me to Scott Peck's remarkable book, *The Road Less Travelled*.

My many spiritual mentors have played an essential guiding role. They have my sincere thanks for their wisdom and their prayers:

- Br George Linnegar, Fr Christopher Channer and Fr Peter Wright, of St Thomas a Becket Church, Lewes.

- Fr Tony Churchill, Deacon John Truman and Fr Christopher Bedford of St Thomas More Church, Seaford.

- Br Francis Edwards, Fr Philip Gaisford and Abbot Christopher Jamison of Worth Abbey.

I am indebted to Patty and Gary Norris, Scott Sollom, Bill Keimig and Fr Richard Cash, visiting tutors at the Maryvale Institute, Birmingham, October 2005, to whom I owe much of my understanding of the need to witness to our own experience of spiritual truths, especially of suffering. They are inspirational teachers.

My thanks should also go to: Ann Bagnall and Dennis Hudson, for advice on presentation and preparation for publishing. Denise Hagger for her kindness in reading the text and offering a potent critique and theological insights. Professor Ian Lewis and Mr Rob Grimer, dedicated consultants in Paediatric Oncology and Orthopaedic Surgery respectively, for their inspirational work and for much of the information in the postscript. Mary and Colin Purchase for their unfailing encouragement and prayers. Rev. Martin Batstone, Chaplain of HM Prison Lewes, for the inspiration of his dedication and care for so many who suffer. For the support of many others, who have often helped without ever knowing it, my heartfelt thanks.

K. A. Allbon, Seaford, July 2008

Introduction

The conjunction of three profound circumstances has led to the writing of this book: my love for Anthony, my godson; the nature of his life and of his passing into new life; the difficult questions, which arose from the tribulation of so many who loved him.

Themes

There are two interwoven strands to this work:

- An account of the life, illness, suffering and death of a child.

- A Christian reflection.

The spiritual reflection arises naturally from the story of Anthony's life and death; in fact, I believe that his sickness and suffering cannot begin to be understood without the light of faith. Thus, the close interweaving of the two strands, which cannot be separated, but whose relative presence in the story will change as it unfolds.

Structure

The book may be divided into three main sections:

- The first three chapters give a summary account of Anthony's brief life, his suffering and death.

- In the central part of the book, the chapters titled Anthony's State of Mind, Superhero, A New Perspective, Behold, Your Mother and The Sleep of Peace consist of a detailed consideration of Anthony's remarkable experiences at the time of his death. The brief but compelling facts are set out and discussed in the form of a speculative analysis in the light of faith. The chapter on Katie is devoted to Katie's revelation of her brother's journey.

- The final two chapters examine the significance of Anthony's life and death and our response to it. We consider his legacy for us and also the difficult questions, doubts and confusions arising from his loss. These reflections are based in the Christian faith.

Assumptions

I have started from the premise that my Christian faith is the only possible approach I can use in considering the mysteries of life and death. Science alone does not get us far; but perhaps the logic of the mind, combined with the vision of the heart, may allow us a slightly fuller appreciation of the value and meaning of Anthony's brief life. I have turned to Scripture for inspiration and for the possible interpretation of some events, spoken words and the inevitable enigmas in this boy's quite remarkable experiences. In doing so I assume – that is, I take for granted – the following:

- The value of each human being is intrinsic and inestimable.

- The Gospels reveal God's purpose for each one of us. He speaks to us here and in many other ways.

- What God says to us may be surprising and it may be life changing, but we shall always recognise His Word as the truth.

Aims.

The book has five objectives:

- A record of Anthony's courageous experience of life, sickness and death.

- To seek an understanding of Anthony's witness to his revelation at the hour of his death.

- The consideration of the questions asked by bereaved families and friends.

- A reflection on these experiences of tribulation as we seek to understand our own lives.

- The opening or reopening of readers' hearts as they grow in love, faith and understanding.

In a sense, the book itself is a journey and the objectives here are the steps taken towards the main aim of the work: I hope that it will be a tribute to Anthony and to all the children and young people who suffer and die so cruelly from cancer and other diseases. Their courage, fortitude, humour and gentle acceptance too often go unrecorded; the tragic loss of families and friends too soon forgotten by the world. But their names, souls, laughter and tears will never die; for God receives them into His glorious protection and reunites them with those they love forever.

Prologue

This account is concerned with a single event in history, unremarkable perhaps in itself, but remarkable to all those connected with it. The event is commonplace enough; the death of an innocent child.

Each year, worldwide, many millions of children die, often in desperate circumstances of disaster, hunger, disease, abuse or neglect. From time to time, our hearts are touched as we see the appalling suffering of children depicted in the media, usually in faraway lands. We do our best, through the many charities, to ease the suffering and our lives move on. It seems to be a commonplace truism that we have to 'get on with our lives', whatever the nature of the tragic events that surround us. Time and again we hear the phrase 'life must go on'. And by and large, in the rich Western world, our comparatively comfortable lives do move on. We put the suffering out of our minds until the next time as we busy ourselves with our daily affairs.

Must life go on as it always did, whatever happens, whatever the cost? What are we alive for? How traumatic do events have to be to cause us to pause, to think, to learn and perhaps even to change direction?

For many parents, families and friends, this point arises when they have to face the suffering and death of a child of their own. This is a suffering from which there is no escape. The death of every child for those who loved and cared for him or her is a life-changing event of often devastating power. The death, which so cruelly claims the child, can maim and stultify many of the surrounding lives.

Such traumatic events, so close to us that they are part of our lives, inevitably force change; change that may be so destructive it may prove impossible for individuals to rebuild any sort of life at all. When the world says 'life must go on', those who have suffered so grievously know that life cannot go on or at the very best it cannot go on with any of the warmth, delight or meaning that once gave it purpose. Quite simply, their hearts are broken. Parents who lose their own children have literally lost the most important part of themselves: physically, emotionally and psychologically, they have lost what they were alive for.

Can any comfort be drawn from such terrible circumstances? What healing can arise from such cruel suffering? What hope have we when we know that death is the inevitable consequence and summation of every human life? The inevitability of death, its unpredictability and our fear of it have made it a taboo subject in our secular Western society. We try not to think of it. But when we lose a person we love, especially a child, we are brought face-to-face with the reality of the human condition. As Thomas More reminds his inquisitors in Robert Bolt's play *A Man for All Seasons*, 'Death … comes for us all, my Lords. Yes, even for Kings he comes.'

No human being can offer definitive answers to the questions raised above, but here and there along life's journey gentle pointers may be discerned. These may lead us in a new direction as we open our eyes to sights, our ears to words and, most importantly, our hearts to truths, which before had remained unknown to us. As we move towards the discovery of these truths, which formerly had been hidden, we approach a treasure, a pearl of great price; an understanding of such momentous value that it is capable of bringing us to a new knowledge of ourselves, a new appreciation of our fellow human beings and a new relationship with the God who created us. We know then that death cannot separate us from those to whom we are bound in love.

The events that have brought me to this conviction concern the suffering and death of my beloved godson Anthony. The circumstances of his death at the age of fifteen are so remarkable and have been so life changing for me, for his parents and for many of those who loved him that it seems imperative to set them down in this record and to consider their significance. For Anthony was able to tell us what was happening to him as he died. The message he has for us is of transforming profundity as he lifts the corner of the veil on the greatest mystery facing each one of us: what is the nature of death and what is the purpose of life?

I have considered Anthony's death and its impact upon me and others in the light of my own evolving faith. In my interpretation of words and events I have made many references to scripture, which has been a guide, a key to the development of understanding and, most importantly, an inexhaustible pool of refreshment for prayer and contemplation.

There is, of course, no other way to examine the central theme considered here. The nature of death, whether of another or, indeed, our own demise to come, is a question not easily examined in our materialistic and secular society. We push it out of our minds, because we neither know how to think about it nor wish to do so. In truth, our society lacks a spiritual dimension. We accept that human beings are mind and body, but when we are faced with the spiritual we draw near unfamiliar territory. For many, this is a lost domain, unapproachable, beyond belief and beyond comprehension.

The loss of the spiritual in our lives is the tragic consequence of our obsession with the material and the intellectual. We think that if we can measure and control things they are real, if we can't they are not. We worship the wrong gods. In our infatuation with ourselves, with individualism, with relativism and with material things, we have lost sight of the important truth that we are made in the image of God. We are mind, body and spirit. Science cannot explain everything; indeed, it gives us little help with our most important questions. We shall only begin to approach an understanding of the mysteries of life and death when we can accept the spiritual dimension within ourselves and within the universe.

Herein lies the key to the exploration of all those questions that arise following the death of a person we love. It is those questions which have prompted this work. In our quest we shall not reach absolute answers, but it is the pathway that matters. For what is life but a journey, a voyage of discovery and preparation, as we move towards a destiny of which we can be certain, but which is seen as through a glass, darkly? (*New Testament*, I Corinthians, 13:12.)

I hope that Anthony's brave journey will offer some consolation to all who suffer in this life and especially to those who have lost their own beloved children, in whatever circumstances. I know that Anthony himself will wish me well in this endeavour and he will reach out his helping hand to all who endure what he and his loved ones have endured.

The Gift of Anthony's Life

Anthony was always seen by his parents Gill and Michael as a joyous gift and an unexpected one. Gill had assumed, on medical advice, that it would be very unlikely that she would have a child. After several years of marriage the couple decided to try for adoption and following the usual formalities and delays, they received into their lives a delightful baby girl, Katie. A short time after Katie's arrival Gill, much to her surprise, became pregnant.

Anthony was born on 28 December 1986 at the Royal Sussex County Hospital, Brighton. The joy of his arrival was tempered somewhat by his illness in infancy, but Ant (as he was to be called by the immediate members of his family) came through his early problems and grew into a happy toddler. At a young age, he showed an observant curiosity about the way the world worked and he was blessed with a naturally friendly nature.

As he grew into his school years, his enquiring mind led him into an exploration of the natural world and of everything scientific, an interest that lasted for all of his short life. This, he combined with an active imagination, expressed in his play and in his model making. He loved creating things, from robots to landscapes and from tanks and soldiers to dinosaurs and imaginary monsters. Ant built small-scale replicas of them all from an early age and he accumulated a vast collection of models and toys which, to his mum's frustration, tended to overflow from his room into every corner of the family home. When his parents brought him to visit me, after a brief 'hello', he would rush upstairs to my 'den'. There, he would work away in contented silence on some new design, using the resources of paper, card and glue available, only to emerge hours later proudly bearing his new creation, which invariably had some operating parts ingeniously worked by systems of pins and card or wire levers.

Anthony was blessed with a gentle personality. He was reserved with strangers, though highly observant of them. Once he knew you and approved of you, he had absolutely no reservations about chattering freely or about expressing his mind; and he certainly knew his own mind. At the same time, he was sensitive and could be hurt by the clumsy or thoughtless remarks of others. Although he was patient with people, he did not suffer fools gladly and would simply ignore those he considered self-obsessed or opinionated. Conversely, Ant felt deeply for those who were disadvantaged in any way or for weaker playmates who appeared to be 'underdogs' with others. At school, he was brave enough to stand by classmates who were unpopular or who were in trouble because they had made silly mistakes. He was loyal to his friends, but made no great demands of them and he accepted them for who they were.

Ant's most outstanding characteristic was his sense of humour. This was ever-present, wry and offbeat, much to the amusement of all who knew him, and it lasted him to the end. His favourite TV programme was *The Simpsons*, which amused him greatly and which he watched at every opportunity. No doubt this egregious and clever series had a certain influence on Ant's already quirky humour. He would chide pomposity and unnecessary seriousness in his elders and he could be a stern critic of his teachers – though keeping his silence until he was home! But kindness, fairness and a concern for those who needed help were qualities of which Anthony approved and which he practised; fortunately, such qualities were to be found in several of his teachers at both his junior and his secondary schools.

Ant was a clever lad, though his attitude to the world was probably too relaxed to mould him into an academic, and he had far too many creative and imaginative interests of his own to want to give too much of his valuable time to school work. As things turned out, he proved his point; life is too short to waste time with the merely routine, the mundane and the mediocre. But, by dint of unusual effort at the age of eleven, Anthony passed the entrance examination to gain a place at Lewes Old Grammar School. Ant had never met a secondary school head before and at his interview he was unexpectedly impressed by the kind and friendly personality of the headmaster Dr Hodd. 'LOGS', as it is affectionately known by all in Lewes, is a small, delightful school with a family atmosphere and a galaxy of individualistic staff and pupils. Into this melange, Anthony fitted perfectly. To him, I think the rambling buildings resembled a sort of mini Hogwarts School; an impression heightened by certain teachers, who were definitely placed by him in a distinctly supernatural category! Despite this he loved them all and he spoke with particular affection of his kindly form master Mr Neil Mitchell, who entrusted him with posting his letters in the little mailbox outside the arched front door of the antiquated main school building. He also held a special regard for his gentle and amusing English and German master Mr John Boyden, with whom his own sense of humour chimed perfectly.

John Boyden is a reserved and studious man who has an intuitive ability as a teacher and he was well loved by his pupils and colleagues. Mr Boyden shared Anthony's particular fondness for *The Simpsons*; its outrageously disrespectful approach to most aspects of life appealed to them both. Anthony and his schoolmates would imitate the unmistakably inane voice and expressions of Homer Simpson in class, hoping that they could get away with it, in full knowledge of John's fondness for the cartoon series. John, secretly amused by this, was loath to put an end to their banter, but their respect for him would claim their attention – at least for the time being. Not long after Anthony's death, John retired from teaching. He told me that his life had been changed by Ant's personality and by his bravery and death. He was, he said, delighted to have known such an amusing and gentle boy; he would never forget him. A kind and generous expression from a gifted teacher, which meant so much to me and to Anthony's family. John's, of course, was not the only heart that Anthony touched and we shall mention several others in the next chapter when we consider his illness.

To his schoolmates, Anthony was known as 'Fish', because of the supposed likeness of his surname, Pilcher, to the tinned variety, pilchards. By coincidence, he was also a very good swimmer. Ant was proud of his nickname; I well remember one occasion, when he was quite small, in his first year at LOGS, attempting to negotiate a crowd of larger boys blocking the school door at 4.00 p.m. He simply said, 'Fish coming through,' at which they good-humouredly parted to let the little lad pass. There is no doubt that Anthony was very happy at this wonderful school, where all the pupils and staff are valued for what they are. It is heartening to know that he spent the last few years of his healthy life in such an enjoyable place. He made many friends at LOGS, but among the best was his classmate Lewis Richardson. Lewis shared many of his interests and he faithfully stood by Anthony through his long illness. Lewis always had Ant's complete trust, a dedication that was reciprocated and has not ceased since Ant's death; for Lewis has an important role in the charity subsequently established in Anthony's memory and he has worked hard with Gill to make it a success. Since leaving school, Lewis has established himself in a fine career in New York. How Anthony would love to be working with him there, for New York was a place he always dreamed of visiting. We shall have cause to mention Lewis again during Anthony's story.

Anthony's concern for another school friend, Daniel, may be cited as an example of his care for classmates who were having difficulties of any kind. Daniel was a lively and intelligent boy, who was not having an easy time at school because of problems at home. He was befriended by Anthony, who was prepared to take risks in his care for, and defence of, the more vulnerable boy. Daniel was a victim of others' as much as of his own mistakes and when he was having problems, Anthony would do his best to explain the lad's case to the school authorities. One morning, they were both in trouble, when Anthony was trying to persuade a disheartened Daniel to walk up to school with him from the railway station. Ant's persuasion worked and they both made it to school, but too late for registration. As a result, both boys had an interview with the head. Anthony was certainly not accustomed to being in trouble, but his explanation of events was accepted by the perceptive headmaster and all was well. It seems that Anthony was able to see into the heart of a troubled friend, whose weaknesses were, at times, exploited and his problems compounded by his less caring fellows. Daniel has since grown into a happy and responsible young man. His affection for Anthony remains (no doubt it will never leave him) and Daniel is earnest in his support of Anthony's cancer charity.

Lewes Old Grammar School was deeply affected by Anthony's illness and death. During his illness, he was far too sick to attend school, but they put on a series of 'Fish Aid' concerts, largely masterminded by Lewis, to raise money for Ant's fledgling bone cancer charity. After he died, the school arranged a moving memorial service for Anthony in St Michael's Church, Lewes. I shall never forget the atmosphere, as the whole school assembled in silence. All had known him, all would miss him and all would remember him. The headmaster's address was a moving tribute to a courageous young man who had been a proud member of a unique and friendly school. His portrait photograph hangs in the corridor of Tyne House as a permanent reminder of his bravery and his love for his school. The headmaster told me that he was particularly fond of the photograph, because Anthony looked so proud of his school uniform. He was proud, indeed, to be part of such a school, where each pupil is valued as a unique individual and is encouraged to develop his or her own gifts.

Anthony lived the whole of his short life in the family home at Peacehaven on the Sussex coast. There is no doubt that he was and is much loved by his family. He was very close to his mum, who was devoted to him. His father, too, loved him dearly and there was an assortment of aunts, uncles, cousins and grandparents all living nearby. His adopted sister Katie was tolerated in outward appearances in a typical brotherly way but, in fact, was dearly loved; though he probably would not have admitted it for fear that the praise should go to her head!

Animals, too, he loved and they loved him. For the last year of his life he had a dear little dog called Toto, bought for him during his illness. She loved Ant and she spent much of his final months snuggling on his bed, a great comfort to him. Before his illness, as I lived in Lewes at the time, I would frequently walk home with Anthony from LOGS at the end of the school day. If we had time we would make a diversion past the ramparts of Lewes Castle, so that Ant could greet a rather large tabby cat named Charlie. He waited for Ant every day at about 4.00 p.m., usually curled up under a public bench, which afforded lovely views over the Sussex Weald from the Castle Mound. Charlie only expected a little stroking and a few words of comfort from his young friend and then he would be content until the next time. I suspect his animal friends must miss dear Anthony at least as much as his human ones.

In view of his later experiences, it should be stated that Anthony was not a particularly religious boy and neither did he show any interest in attending church regularly. He had been baptised and he had enjoyed Sunday school in his younger years, but his Christian education seems to have been limited to what he had been taught there and at school. He was brought up in the secular lifestyle fairly typical of Britain in the late twentieth century. Though a young scientist by ability and inclination, he accepted with interest the probability of a supernatural world over and above the material universe and he was intrigued to ponder over the nature and power of God as a divine creator. He enjoyed considering and discussing such matters. It is possible that they may have influenced the sense of justice and kindness that was a characteristic feature of his personality.

Anthony possessed a quality of innocence, in the sense that for him, things were often obvious in a simple, direct way that they were not for many others. His guileless acceptance of his way of seeing things could give him a quite remarkable force of conviction. He was sometimes surprised to find that others lacked this straightforward persuasion, because for them the world was more complex, their view less certain. In a sense, this gave Anthony a degree of vulnerability. In his honest candour he could be hurt by the inability of others to appreciate what he saw as his own clarity of vision. But Anthony's insight endowed him with a sense of resolution and thus strength of personality not so common in one of his age. Though blessed with an innocence of spirit, he was not naive and his decisive character combined with his sharp sense of humour made him a valuable classmate. His friends recognised his independent perception and they knew that he could be an intriguing and questioning companion.

Anthony always accepted absolutely the authority, learning and judgement of his teachers. He placed his complete trust in them. At times, he was disappointed to discover that they were only human. His grandad related to me an amusing example of this, when Ant was a small boy at infants' school. It was sports day and eventually the time came for the boys' race. They lined up enthusiastically; each determined to prove himself to his proud, onlooking parents. The boys made ready to run and as a hush fell over the assembled crowd, the teacher in charge called, 'Ready, steady, go.' And they were off … all but Ant! He stood at the starting line with a look of mixed perplexity and disappointment. When his grandad asked him why he had not started with the other boys, Anthony replied in bewilderment, 'But she told us we were only to run when she said, "One, two, three, off" – she didn't say it!' Anthony expected absolute consistency from adults in authority – he frequently did not get it. He began to learn the ways of the world.

When Anthony was four, his parents, whose relationship had been deteriorating, decided to divorce. The children thereafter lived with their mother, but frequently visited their father, who moved to a flat only a mile or two away. Thus, an event all too common in our society overtook this family. As in so many examples of separation and divorce, we do not know what the effect on the children may have been, but they appeared to cope with it. Eventually, after a few years, Michael, Ant's father, was to remarry. Just before this event, as Katie, Ant and I walked along the street, I recall Anthony asking me a question in his normal, straightforward way. 'Do you like kittens, Ken?' 'Yes,' I said. 'Well, that's all right then,' came the reply, 'cos Dad's going to give Katie and me a kitten each. It's all part of the package.' Ant's wonderfully matter-of-fact approach to an event that was changing their lives so profoundly was typical. He did not let the affairs of the world around him impinge too much on his equanimity. The resilience of childhood seemed to carry Katie and Anthony through, but we shall never know what they might have suffered at that time, when they were so young.

Thus, Anthony began his short life. In many ways it was unremarkable, but perhaps it was not ordinary. Though, like most children, Ant had his trying moments, he was a much loved and loving boy. Intelligent, gentle, sensitive and imaginative, by the time he started his teenage years he was about as far removed from a 'young thug' as could be imagined. Anthony brought joy to many and, as his headmaster was to say of him on a later occasion, 'He seemed to spread a sense of light and warmth to those around him.' Praise, indeed, and confirmation of the wonderful gift that was Anthony's life. A life so full of promise that was to be so short. Was the promise of his life unrealised? Or was the realisation of this gentle, young life already there to be seen by eyes that see? Now we look back with the advantage of hindsight, do we sense what we might have appreciated so much more fully at the time?

The deeper meanings of life often seem to be paradoxical and we have to consider the paradox of gifts given and taken back again. How can we, who have loved a child, come to any sort of acceptance of the fact that this gift, such a wonderful gift, the gift that was our heart's delight and a gift so freely and unexpectedly given, can be taken away again with such cruel abruptness? What are we to make of a world in which the promises of a loving God are apparently overwhelmed on every side by the inexorable and unforeseeable rule of death?

It is probable that God gives us gifts, not for ourselves, but for others. We accept His wonderful gifts, too often taking them for granted, only to find that they are not ours to possess, after all. We have to ask ourselves questions about what we can possess of value in the world, about the meaning of possession and its importance to us.

It seems that we want to possess so many things in perpetuity; our own survival and security and that of those we love, the love and affirmation we receive from others and our ability to have power – to control our lives and those of the people we need. We assume that we have a right to all these things and more, as well as to all our material possessions. Somehow, these are needs we cannot do without. We forget that a large part of the world's population lives in poverty, misery, disease and starvation. These are the places where the loss of a child is commonplace. Where we have gifts we are lucky, indeed. If any gift is taken from us, many are they who never had such a gift or from whom everything has been taken.

We must live for the moment and learn to give of our gifts; to give freely to others as we have been given; to accept joyfully what God has chosen for us and to respond with kindness and love. We must learn to see time as an irrelevance. A beautiful life on this earth, however short, will live on into eternity. Those with a long and selfish life, grasping to hang on to every security, every affirmation, every source of power and wealth, will lose everything. Jesus makes this quite clear to us when He is talking to the multitude at Caesarea Philippi:

> For whoever would save his life will lose it;
> and whoever loses his life for my sake and the
> gospel's will save it.
> For what does it profit a man,
> to gain the whole world and forfeit his life?
>
> (Mark 8:35–36.)

The gift God gives us is His love. It is all we need and it comes to us in so many ways, especially in those we love. In this world, death will come for them eventually and also for us. But the love we have received and given endures and it is the source of all hope. It is this love that goes beyond all the world has to offer, into a new and glorious reality.

In the tribulation of our lives, Christ constantly reassures us, 'Be not afraid.' It is a promise, which will be fulfilled. Its implications are astounding, not least for the lives of the beloved children we believe have been taken from us. In truth, we have not lost them, for here on earth they live on in our hearts and in the world to come we shall be reunited with them forever.

Sickness and Suffering

Towards the end of his second year at Lewes Old Grammar School, in the summer of 2000, Anthony fell awkwardly on the pavement outside of school while carrying his heavy school bag full of books. He hurt his left knee quite badly and took some time to recover from this trauma.

During the early part of his third year at the school, the same knee once again started to give him pain. His mum said that that each time they visited the GP, the 'cause' always seemed to be some accidental trauma, such as being hit by a football or being inadvertently kicked in games or in the playground.

Eventually, the GP sent a request for an urgent referral to the orthopaedic consultant at the Royal Alexandra Hospital for Sick Children, Brighton. Before the date for his appointment came through, Anthony was by now in so much pain that his nanny (his maternal grandmother), who had an appointment to see a chiropractor, took him to the hospital with her. The date of this visit was Tuesday, 3 April 2001. The chiropractor was so concerned when she saw Ant that she took X-rays of his leg. That evening, she called Gill to let her know there was a problem. She had established that Anthony had a tumour on the lower end of the left femur, just above the knee, and so she sent them straight to the accident and emergency department at Royal Sussex County Hospital. Anthony was diagnosed with osteosarcoma (primary bone cancer) on 4 April 2001. The correct diagnosis had taken six months since he first complained of pain in his knee in October 2000; we were later to become aware that late diagnosis is commonplace in this very dangerous cancer of children and young people. Ant was 14 years old and he was quite a small lad for his age. What he lacked in size he more than made up for in courage over the coming months. His mum said that from that day on, their lives changed completely. They were never to return to normal.

Within five days Anthony and Gill had visited four different hospitals; Gill said that they were well treated and they found all the staff to be efficient, friendly and caring. They were told that the survival rates from the initial tumour for non-metastasised patients (i.e. where the cancer has not spread) are about sixty per cent in the UK and for those with metastasis only thirty per cent are likely to survive. The tumour, we were assured, was quite unrelated to the original fall, when Anthony had first hurt his left knee. While accepting the wisdom of the medical experts, we have continued to be a little uncertain about this, particularly since Gill was to discover that many other children with osteosarcoma seem to have experienced previous trauma in the affected area.

The first of a gruelling round of hospital visits that were to continue for the rest of his life was to the Royal National Orthopaedic Hospital, Stanmore, 17–20 April 2001 and it was here that initial tests were completed. On Ant's second visit to Stanmore on 22–23 April, there were yet more tests and a biopsy operation. In this process, a small sample of the tumour is removed, so that the consultant can diagnose the tumour type and determine the most appropriate chemotherapy treatment. This has to be done before the tumour is affected by chemotherapy.

On Friday, 27 April, at the Royal Marsden Hospital, Sutton, the nature of his disease and his forthcoming treatment was explained to Anthony in great detail by the consultant, Professor Pinkerton. This compassionate consultation was heartbreaking to behold. The learned doctor, as kind and gentle as he was clever, sat next to Ant on the edge of his bed, with his arm tenderly round the boy's shoulder. Anthony listened in rapt attention as he came to understand the gravity of the quiet words he was hearing. Silent tears flooded the usually bright eyes we loved so much. The anguish in the room was palpable as we witnessed this gentle boy, who had done none harm and thought none harm, coming to the realisation that his life was to be disrupted for the foreseeable future and that over his future there hung the most appalling question mark.

To me, this initial horror of Anthony's coming to an understanding of his cruel and undeserved fate was the most poignant and disturbing episode in the long saga of his suffering. For a child, it was surely too much to endure. But Ant came through it with immense courage and, at the end, he found his consolation in the loving arms of his mum as their tears and love flowed freely. On this day, both Gill and Anthony's hearts were broken, but in their anguish, the immensity of their love was sealed forever. Through my own tears, as I beheld this suffering and love, there was a glimpse of the reality beyond the world; for I was witness to the true value and meaning of human life. I knew that I was never so honoured and never so proud as to have been chosen as godfather to this wonderful, courageous boy.

Anthony was told that he had osteosarcoma in the form of a localised, malignant tumour, growing on the lower outside of the left femur. Although rare (there are about 400 cases of primary bone cancer in the UK each year), it usually affects children and young adults. Often, it is the legs that are afflicted, but sometimes the arms. The symptoms are local swelling and increasing pain. Over the course of treatment, the pain would be controlled by drugs. In Anthony's case, the cancer did not seem to have metastasised. Osteosarcoma, however, is a rather aggressive cancer, which tends to spread to other bones or to the lungs. Eventually, Anthony would have two tubes inserted into his body. The first was a Hickman Line, in the form of a clear plastic tube, inserted directly into his chest to allow the intravenous supply of drugs, including the chemotherapy drugs. The Hickman Line also allowed blood transfusions to be given when required. Later, as he lost weight through failing to eat because of nausea induced by chemotherapy, a gastrostomy tube, formed from a similar plastic pipe, was passed into his stomach, so that he could be fed directly when he felt too sick to eat or drink.

Anthony was to be given two chemotherapy drugs. The aim of these was to reduce the tumour by destroying all the dividing cells in the body. This meant that his growth would be interrupted, but would resume after treatment. It was explained that these powerful drugs would have serious side effects and that both of them would cause nausea and vomiting. In addition, a rare side effect of the drug cisplatin was that it could affect the hearing and the kidneys. The second drug, doxorubicin, would suppress bone marrow growth (thus, the need for transfusions of blood and platelets) and it would cause red urine, a sore mouth and temporary hair loss. It could also affect the heart, but this was rare.

The chemotherapy would consist of a six-month course, starting on 3 May 2001, and it would take place at the Royal Marsden Hospital. During this time, there would be three weeks on, followed by three weeks off the drugs; i.e. four cycles of chemotherapy treatment. As things turned out, Ant reacted so badly to the drugs that he took longer and longer in the recovery phases between each of the 'chemo' treatments. In the end, he had six cycles of treatment in all.

Anthony would undergo surgery to remove the tumour, along with the bones of the entire knee joint. A metal (titanium) prosthesis would be inserted to replace the joint. This operation would be done after the size of the tumour had been reduced by two cycles of chemotherapy. Radiotherapy (using X-rays) would not be part of Ant's treatment; we were told that sometimes this is used as an alternative to surgery. The surgery would be done at the Royal National Orthopaedic Hospital and the consultant surgeon was to be Mr Briggs.

Anthony's first chemotherapy cycle at the Royal Marsden Hospital was done during the period 3–7 May. He reacted very badly to the chemotherapy, which made him extremely nauseous and as a result he could not face eating more than a mouthful or so of food at each meal. This caused rapid weight loss and increasing weakness. Ant began to take on a pale and skeletal appearance, though he was quite amused to think that he probably looked like an alien being from another world. Indeed, his sense of humour never deserted him, even in the depths of his adversity, and he did his best to make little of his suffering. His mum told me of one such amusing incident, which occurred shortly after they had returned home from a 'chemo' session at the Marsden. Anthony sat in his hospital bed in the living room, hunched over his sick basin (he called it his 'sick bucket') in the midst of a bout of violent nausea. It happened that his nanny chose this moment to enter the room clutching a glass of wine. He did not fail to notice the wine and with head still down and retching loudly, he reached out his free arm in a mock demand for the glass. Ant's humour was a bright gift, lifting the exhausted spirits of those who cared for him so desperately.

To help Anthony's intake of nourishment, the gastrostomy tube was inserted into his stomach on 29 May. On the next day, he started the second cycle of chemotherapy, again reacting badly, as proved always to be the case with this aggressive therapy. There was some concern that he might be too weak for the surgery, now due to take place, to remove the tumour. Eventually, the operation was done at Stanmore on Wednesday, 27 June. The procedure was a long and complex one and it was additionally stressful for Anthony and his family, because they were told that if things went wrong during the operation, the surgeons may have no option but to amputate the leg. The weak little lad went into the operating theatre, together with his favourite Pikachu bear, not knowing whether he would emerge with both legs intact.

As things turned out, all seemed to go well and when he awoke from the anaesthetic he was relieved to see that he still had both legs, even though, of course, there was no feeling in his left leg for some time. Unfortunately, however, the new prosthetic joint caused him considerable trouble and pain. It was never to work properly and, as a result, he had only a limited degree of flexibility in his left leg. Also, he never recovered full sensation in his lower leg and his foot dropped rather badly. He was not able to walk again without the aid of crutches and then only for short distances, as he was too weak for sustained effort. It was hoped that Anthony would regain enough strength to allow a second operation, with the intention of restoring full mobility to his knee joint. Sadly, as Anthony declined, there was never time for this to be carried out.

Following surgery, it was deemed necessary for Ant to have four more cycles of chemotherapy. He completed the treatment on 17 December 2001 and on Friday, 28 December it was Anthony's birthday. He was 15 years old and although we did not know it at the time, it was to be his last birthday. Anthony had always loved this time of year, around Christmas and his birthday, and this year they were blended together into one long celebration. Fortunately, he was well enough to enjoy this happy time and to revel in the large number of presents with which he was indulged.

During the period from September to December 2001, in the 'recovery' stages between chemo cycles, Ant enjoyed some other happy times. He had asked his mum in April, after their first visit to the Royal Marsden Hospital, if it would be possible to raise money for bone cancer research, so that other children might not have to go through what he was about to endure. The first money came in when he was sponsored to have his head shaved (before he lost his hair during chemo). Later, more money was raised by his school at 'Fish Aid' concerts, largely organised by Anthony's friend and schoolmate Lewis. On Wednesday, 26 September, Ant was able to visit the school in his wheelchair, to receive a cheque from the headmaster for £750. Eventually, the charity funds were to grow and the charity itself was to evolve into the Anthony Pilcher Bone Cancer Trust. (The development of the Charity is outlined in the postscript.)

One of Anthony's favourite hobbies had been building and painting the models for the Games Workshop Group Plc. war-games. Each September, the Games Workshop holds a major exhibition of new products at the National Exhibition Centre in Birmingham. For the South Coast contingent of devotees, a coach is organised from Brighton to Birmingham, leaving early in the morning and returning the same evening. Ant had been hoping that he would be well enough to go. Fortunately, he was strong enough and Lewis, always a stalwart friend, took charge of the wheelchair and complete responsibility for Anthony's welfare. They had a wonderfully enjoyable day on Sunday, 30 September, managing to obtain a preview look around all the exhibits because of Ant's wheelchair-bound status. They arrived home completely exhausted, having spent all their pocket money and more.

On 6 October, Ant received a very special present, when his little puppy Toto arrived. She was the double of the small dog in the classic film *The Wizard of Oz*. Toto and Ant loved one another from the start and the little dog must have given him great comfort during the long periods when he was bed-bound, as she happily spent hours curled up with him.

Gill organised a visit to the London Eye on 4 December for Anthony and members of the family. A minibus was hired for the day, which proved to be a great success. Anthony was delighted by the fact that the great wheel had to be brought to a complete stop to allow his wheelchair to be pushed carefully into the car. Once installed, he was granted the place of honour in the nose cone of the 'viewing module'. The views were particularly impressive in the mid-afternoon of that memorable December day as the sun started to sink down over west London. It was a happy day and evening, rounded off by a fine pub supper on the way home. Ant had entered into the festive occasion by wearing his Father Christmas hat and he was in good spirits, though rather tired as we made the final stage of the journey home.

Throughout this period, Anthony's health was steadily declining, but in fits and starts. There would be periods of several days when he was too weak to leave his bed, followed by days when he was well enough to be up and perhaps able to do some model-making or painting. Increasingly frequent visits were made to the children's hospital in Brighton (the Royal Alexandra) for transfusions of blood or platelets, needed because the drug doxorubicin had stopped his bone marrow from producing new blood cells.

Sometimes, on his better days, when the weather was fair, his mum would take Anthony for a little excursion in his wheelchair. On one such occasion, when I was with them, a minor but telling encounter occurred as we meandered slowly along the estate roads. On the surface of events it is scarcely memorable but, in fact, redolent with hidden meaning and truth. Ant was snug in his wheelchair, well wrapped up by his mum against the coastal breeze so prevalent in Peacehaven. The street was quiet, but as we walked along, we became aware of three or four youths approaching on the opposite pavement. They had a rough and ready appearance, with a lively walk and hoods up against the cool air; probably not a group of boys Ant would have expected even to notice him. As they neared us, they became aware of Anthony and crossed the road to approach his wheelchair. Although strangers, they greeted him in earnest friendliness.

'Hello, matey. How are you doing?' said one.

'Are you alright today, mate?' asked another.

Ant, no doubt surprised by this unexpected salutation of kindness, replied quietly, 'Yes, thank you very much.'

'Take care then, mate. See you soon,' said the boys, as with friendly smiles and nods of farewell they continued on their way.

These lads, who could readily have been regarded as 'yobs' (and were no doubt absent from school) had recognised Anthony's disadvantaged situation and, to our surprise, had taken the trouble to give him some kind words of encouragement. Their completely spontaneous and unexpected support must have been as heartening to Ant as it was to his mum and to me. May God bless those boys for their touching concern; they probably did not realise the power of the humanity they had shown in those few moments.

Into the New Year, 2002, Anthony's slow, downward path continued. At Christmas 2001 the new film *The Fellowship of the Ring* had come out, the first in the sequence of *The Lord of the Rings* films. Ant was very keen to see this amazing fantasy, which included some of the characters he'd had the opportunity to paint as miniature Games Workshop models. In late January, he was well enough and I was able to take him to the cinema at Brighton Marina on the twenty-third. Wheelchair access was no problem and there was a designated space at the rear of the cinema from where we could watch in comfort. He very much enjoyed the experience and I think he felt that it was the best film he had ever seen. He may have changed his mind later in the year, for we were able to make one more visit to the cinema in June. This will be recounted in the next chapter.

The date of Katie's eighteenth birthday was 8 March 2002. First, a party for all the family and friends was arranged in a hired hall for Saturday, 2 March. It was a joyful event and Anthony was able to attend in his wheelchair. It was adorned with an 'L' plate, because Lewis was the driver for the evening. On Friday, 8 March, the family enjoyed dinner at a restaurant in Seaford. Much to Katie's delight, Ant was able to be there to complete the party. He sat at the head of the table, to allow sufficient space for his wheelchair. Unfortunately, because of his poor appetite, he was not able to do justice to most of the tasty food available.

Throughout his illness, Anthony only once asked, 'Why me?' He never complained and he kept his sense of humour throughout his ordeal. Everyone who helped him or who had contact with him at this time, especially his nurses and doctors, remembers him for his strong personality and his cheeky sense of fun. When he was not in hospital, Anthony was looked after at home by his mum and by a team of visiting nurses and doctors. A nurse usually visited each day to keep a careful check on him and a hospital bed had been set up in the living room for the convenience of Ant and his many visitors. As I lived nearby, I was lucky enough to be able to see him frequently and we had many interesting conversations. Sometimes, we would attempt a little school work and on other occasions we enjoyed watching one of his favourite films on video.

During one such visit we touched upon the subject of death. We had rarely spoken of it, though by the time of this conversation it seemed possible that Ant may not live much longer. He accepted this with equanimity and he was quite certain that he would 'be in Heaven'. I think, in his usual enquiring way, he was intrigued to consider what it might be like there. He said, 'Anyway, Ken, one day, before too long, you will join me there.' I told him that it was good of him to think so, but there was a slight problem, because I might have some difficulty in getting past St Peter at the Pearly Gates. 'Don't be silly, Ken,' said Ant, 'I'll keep my foot in the door for you!' What wonderful faith from my dear godson. It seems that his guidance of me in spiritual matters was far greater than any such help I was able to offer him in my role as godfather. This was but an early indication that the experience and the words of this child were to be nothing short of life changing for those close to him.

Anthony's suffering during his illness was appalling to see. He lost so much weight and was so weak that he became still further a ghostly silhouette of his former self, a faint outline, scarcely recognisable. This, however, was typical of most of the other child cancer patients I saw when visiting Ant in hospital. As I am sure it has to many others, my first visit to the Royal Marsden Hospital came as a harrowing shock to me. The vision of the rows of cots occupied by sweet children, reduced to skeletal ghosts yet still smiling, was a haunting sight. It was redolent only of those appalling immediate post-war revelations at such camps of horror as Belsen and Auschwitz. Like them, it is a vision one can never lose. The difference is that these children are being well looked after; the malady does not come from those responsible for them, but from elsewhere. The wonderful staff who deal with these terribly sick children at the Royal Marsden, the 'Royal Alex' and many similar hospitals are motivated by compassion and kindness and their actions are carried through by skill, bravery and dedication beyond belief. The reward they get for their compassion comes from the frail beauty, the sweet, sad love of the children in their care and from the grateful dependence of the shattered, exhausted parents, whose hearts are broken, lives ruined and who have nowhere else to turn. The world gives these wonderful nurses and doctors no due recognition for what they do. How can it? It is too busy 'getting on with life'. What they do and what arises from their compassion is on a different plane, a higher plane, that transcends the normal values of the world. In our blinkered society, perhaps it is as well that all this sadness and all this wonder is safely out of the way behind the hospital walls.

I know that many of the friends that Anthony made during this time of suffering, nurses, doctors and fellow patients, were very important to him. He was sustained and strengthened by these warm relationships. There were so many of them. I remember Keith from Folkestone, a pleasant boy of the same age as Ant, with exactly the same illness, who lay in the bed next to him at Stanmore. Unlike Ant, Keith was a great sportsman, so the loss of his mobility must have been doubly shattering. Their commiserations and friendly chatter were certainly of great mutual support. Sadly, Keith was to die a little before Ant.

Without doubt, Anthony's favourite nurse at the Royal Alex was Kara. She loved him dearly and was greatly loved in return. Her kindness, her gentle care and her wonderful smile were a rich treasure, a source of warmth and affirmation in his weakness. Fortunately, Gill was able to take Ant in his wheelchair to Kara's wedding on 27 July 2002, only a couple of months before he died. This must have meant so much to him, for Kara's sustaining love will never leave Anthony's heart. Kara is blessed with a little son of her own now, Joseph; he could not want for a better mum.

Another nurse inseparable from Anthony's story is Francis, a community nurse who visited Ant when he was in bed at home, between hospital sessions. Francis also formed a very warm relationship with Ant and it left him with a special sense of peace, calm and refreshment after every visit. Anthony had enormous respect for Francis and he trusted him completely. That trust was founded in Francis' skill and his goodness, a goodness based on a life of prayer. His prayers, and those of his community at Worth Abbey, brought Anthony a peace the world alone cannot give.

Beryl, a nurse from Crossroads, also visited at home. Her sense of humour was as sharp as Ant's and they had some wonderful, warm-hearted, verbal sparring sessions. She rejoiced in singing while she worked but, after the first brave attempts in Ant's hearing, was forbidden in no uncertain terms to do so again! Despite the threat of her warbling, Ant and Toto both found great fun in Beryl's visits and she had Anthony's heartfelt confidence. Shortly after his death, she told me that the dear little chap had confided in her a week or two earlier. He had told her that one of his saddest regrets was that he would never know what it was like to be married. The poignancy and earnestness of this was heartbreaking, she said. The poor boy knew that he was dying, of course, and it was one of the few regrets he expressed, that he was to be denied some of the fullness of life. Beryl told me that in her long experience as a paediatric nurse, this was one of the most touching moments she had ever had. He was an innocent child, who had never become a teenager in his body; furthermore, his poor body lay wasted and frail before her as he imparted this sad confidence with a trust that implied complete love. She was, she said, honoured to have known him and to have cared for him. She will never forget him.

Although Ant's body was halted in its development by the appalling grip of his disease and its aggressive treatment, his mental and emotional development followed the opposite course. While retaining his humorous and pleasant personality, he was accelerated from childhood to manhood in his disposition and understanding. His integrity, strength of character and intuitive understanding of others came to a fruition not normally seen before mature adulthood. This transformation of Anthony's maturity was rapid and it was remarked on by his mum. He seemed to grow through the suffering he endured into a complete person, while retaining the delightful and humorous candour, which marked his childhood. We beheld an enigma; as his body was ruined by disease, his inner self rapidly blossomed before us. He was denied fullness in his physical being as he embraced the fullness of life and understanding we would expect to be the rare blessing of many years. In his sickness, Ant showed us that true health is understanding – mental, moral and spiritual. It is the gift of wisdom, rarely granted to men or women. Where Anthony's gift would lead us, had yet to be revealed.

During his last few months, Gill took Anthony from time to time to a faith healer called Linda Green. Linda's relaxing therapy was able to bring him a wonderful sense of calm. After each visit he came away with renewed strength and peace, enabling him once again to face the struggles of his daily routine. I know, too, that Gill gained much supportive strength from Linda's restorative healing.

All these people and so many more sustained Anthony's morale during the final months of his life. But, as with any child, he drew his strength, security and his affirmation as a person from his parents. They formed him as an individual and it was to them that he owed his first love. Ant's greatest source of strength was his mum. Gill's love for her son was as incredible as any mother's love could be. She had carried him with delight, after quite an unexpected conception, for she believed she could have no children. She had brought him into the world and he was her only natural child. She suffered grievously during Anthony's illness, but for those terrible eighteen months she was with him day and night, both in hospital and at home. She was exhausted, but every day, again and again, Gill found the strength to keep going. She would never leave his side; Ant knew his beloved mum was always there for him, whenever he opened his eyes.

Ant and his mum had made a pact between them as their hearts broke in the agony of their mutual grief. They agreed that they would shed their tears together – supporting one another in their common love and grief. In this way, the tears that were born out of their love belonged only to them. They hoped, also, to spare their many visitors the tears of their suffering, for they knew that much braveness was needed by those who came to see them in love. I can scarcely think of a tenderer image, summing up the mystery of this dear boy's illness, than that of Gill and Anthony, mother and son, crying softly together as they hugged each other, warmly enfolded in their love. I am certain of the tears shed by God himself as His invisible presence filled their hearts.

The sense of love between Anthony and Gill was palpable. As he faded in his last weeks, that sense strengthened and as he fell into his final sleep, he was in her loving arms and he would not have wished for more than that.

Gill's loss was incalculable. No one, of course, can understand the depth of her suffering. With the greatest love comes the greatest suffering. No one in this world can offer her any recompense. Only those who have lost children in similar circumstances can hope to form a bond of support in their mutual grief. Gill has drawn strength from her friendship with her namesake Gill Callar from Cornwall, who sadly lost her daughter Emma to the same disease at about the same time. Together, and with the help of many other parents who have also suffered the loss of children to this terrible cancer, they now work hard to raise money to further research and understanding in a neglected area of oncology. Their love for their children will never die and they continue to labour in their children's names and memories to reduce childhood suffering in the future.

Michael, Anthony's father, loved his only son dearly and now during the boy's suffering was disadvantaged by his work and by his divorce from Gill. He did his best to be with his son, but inevitably the time they could spend together was less than he hoped. Nevertheless, it was doubly valuable for all that and it was time to be richly savoured and well used. Ant's illness brought them together and when Michael's son died, he did so in the certainty of his dad's love. Michael's loss has changed him and brought him a new and fearless understanding of death. The bravery and love of his dear son will always be with him in his heart as an abiding source of strength.

Anthony was very close to his grandparents George and June, Gill's parents, who lived nearby and who provided her with constant support.

It was June, as we have seen, who by taking Ant to the chiropractor ensured the correct diagnosis of his illness. And it was she who took expert care of Katie and Toto, when Gill and Ant were away in hospital, often for long periods. Katie loved being with her nanny and Ant would have trusted his beloved Toto to no one but his nan or his mum. George was a retired bus and coach driver, who befriended everybody. A typical Londoner, with a wonderful sense of humour, he would chatter away to anyone he met and was much regarded by all who knew him. Anthony's sense of humour and his non-stop chatter to those he knew came from George, as did his delight in quizzing family and friends as to their retention and understanding of the latest information (usually about Games Workshop models, or 'superheroes') that he had imparted. We were expected to regard this as 'homework' to be remembered in detail. Needless to say, the results of our frequent verbal tests were invariably low in score! Anthony despaired of us as his pupils, but did not give up – at least, not while his strength lasted. When Anthony died, George had lost one of his best pals and, sadly, he survived his grandson by only two and a half years. Like Ant, he is sorely missed by the many who loved him. George's mortal remains are alongside those of his beloved grandson, in the beautiful garden at The Downs Crematorium, Brighton.

Anthony was called upon to suffer almost beyond endurance during the last eighteen months of his short life. Where did he get the strength to carry him through his afflictions? He was not a big lad, he was not strong physically and he was not aggressive in any way. He was a gentle soul. But he was brave, and immensely so. His courage and humour carried him through to the end, without complaint or self-pity. He knew what was happening to him at every stage. He wanted to know and he accepted it, faced it and just got on with it. How can a child do such a thing? From the strength of his personality we might suppose. Certainly, but at such a time how was his strength sustained? Why did it come and from where?

It came because he was blessed. Blessed by the unceasing dedication of his mum. Blessed by the love of his dad, who also grieved for him and came to see him whenever he could escape from work. Blessed by the love of his family and friends, particularly his grandparents, his nurses, doctors and carers and his school friends, especially Lewis, who stood by him to the end. Blessed by the love of God, who is the author of all love – Anthony rested secure in this love. It affirmed him and it sustained him through his difficulties and his pain. And it worked the other way round, too, as Ant reflected all this love in the light and warmth he showed for those around him. If you were Anthony's friend you helped him in that affirmation, you supported him as he faced his difficulties, just as his gentle spirit was, and still is, there for you.

The bringer of another, and quite unexpected, source of help for Anthony was Kit Wood. Kit was, and still is, a highly respected teacher at Ant's school and he is a man of great kindness. Much moved by the boy's illness, Kit brought for him a small bottle of holy water from Lourdes. He had recently visited the shrine of Our Lady there with a sick friend and had thought the water might bring some blessing and peace to Ant. It was typically kind of him to do this, but he was hesitant to pass it on to the lad, in case he might not appreciate it. Far from it. Anthony loved the little bottle of holy water. It stood on his bedside table from then on and he would not let anyone move it away. With absolute faith, he would carefully remove the cork from the bottle each day and place a little drop of water on his forehead. This was very touching to see, because he was so serious and matter-of-fact about this little ritual. It was a vision of childhood faith. I know that he appreciated so much that Kit had thought about him with such kindness. There is little doubt that Ant was brought much relief at his final time of trial and we are not to know how much the prayers of all those who loved him, combined with the efficacy of the holy water, were contributory to that. As we shall see, those with faith might well suggest that the influence of Mary, the Mother of Christ, was to be profound at the hour of Anthony's death.

As Anthony lay in his bed hour after hour, his weakness increased and only he knew the agony he had to bear, though he did not tell us of this. Fortunately, he was able to sleep for long periods. It seems likely that God, in His love, would have brought him some comfort and solace, perhaps in his dreams. An intimation of this comes from quite an unsolicited remark he made to me one day as I sat at his bedside.

'Ken,' he said, 'you know the angel of death; you know how he is always shown, how he is supposed to be; a horrible old man with a black cloak and hood, the face of a skull and carrying a large, curved blade?'

'You mean a scythe,' I said.

'Yes, that's it,' he went on. 'Well, they have got it wrong. That's not right at all. He is young, very beautiful, all in white and not frightening, but very kind.'

That was all he said. Typically, it was done in his usual matter-of-fact way. I did not press him for any more details. He did not need to give me any. He never mentioned his angel again.

I do not think for a moment that Ant made up this astounding revelation. Why would he need to do any such thing? The fact that such an unusual topic of conversation came out of the blue and was related blandly in his normal factual way is testimony to the truth. It could have arisen from a dream, of course, and thus from the unconscious mind. But from what he said, it seems likely either that Anthony may be right in his view of the angel of death (i.e. we have 'got it wrong') or that the figure he saw was not the bringer of death, but an angel of compassion, who came to comfort him. Either way, we may ask how he was so certain of the angel's kindness. Perhaps Anthony's confidence on this point suggests that the angel actually spoke to him. We shall never know. Anyway, the visitation had a beneficent effect, for it dismissed from his mind the terrible, conventional image of the 'grim reaper', which may well have been troubling him.

Months later, following Ant's death, I was reading about the visions of the children at Fatima in Portugal, in 1916/17. I was struck by the remarkable similarity between Ant's angel and the angel described by the Fatima children. These children said they saw a young man of about 14 to 16 years of age, of extreme beauty. He seemed to be both whiter than snow and as transparent as crystal when the sun shines through it. He told the children not to be afraid and he prayed with them, kneeling down with his head bowed low. Then he disappeared as mysteriously as he had arrived. The similarity with Anthony's angel is striking: young, beautiful, clothed in white, kind and reassuring. The children knew he was kind, because he had spoken to them; perhaps this reinforces our speculation about Ant's confidence in the kindness of his angel. The Fatima angel seems to have come to prepare the children for the vision of Mary they were to have in 1917. Perhaps Anthony's benign visitor came to prepare him for his approaching transition from this world to the next. The events at Fatima will impinge again on Anthony's story.

Throughout this period of his life we can do no other than to draw strength from Anthony's brave example. We learn from him that the end of life in this world is not to be feared. He was not afraid of his approaching death. The song he chose as the retiring music for his own funeral was *Follow Me* by Uncle Kracker. With his typical tongue-in-cheek humour, he reminds us that where he has gone we must follow; there is no other way. One day, we shall all have to follow him as he 'swims through our veins like a fish in the sea'. The music is fun and the words of the song are moving and heartening. Those of the first verse and the chorus are particularly appropriate to Anthony.

The words are full of the truth of Anthony's very being. He could not have chosen a better song to bring the warmth of his presence into the chapel on the tragic day of his funeral. Remarkably, even his nickname 'Fish' brings us the striking conviction that he will continue to occupy the very fabric of our being. In this wonderful little song Anthony warmly encourages us not to be afraid as we prepare to follow him one day. We are to follow his example, for Jesus tells us, 'Whoever humbles himself like this child, he is the greatest in the kingdom of heaven.' (Matt 18:4.) The circumstances of Anthony's death will, by the grace of God, lead us a little further into the mystery of suffering and love and Anthony's request, 'Follow me', will astound us as we tread in his footsteps to the gateway of eternity. The same request is used by our Lord many times in the Gospels. It is worth repeating His succinct recapitulation of His teaching:

> If any man would come after me, let him deny himself
> and take up his cross and *follow me*.
>
> (Mark 8:34.)

Anthony's Death

For the many months since the surgery on his leg Anthony had been confined to his wheelchair. He could only walk a few painful steps on his crutches and, as the weeks passed, he became weaker and more restricted to his bed. For a period, he was given steroids to increase his weight. This, they did, but at the cost of unpleasant side effects, including the fattening out of his face, so that for a time his appearance changed for all those who knew him.

On 20 April 2002, a routine check showed that the cancer had spread to both of Anthony's lungs and it was inoperable. This was devastating news, the implications of which were inevitable. We knew now that Ant's brave fight against his cruel disease was all but over. On 2 May, he started a different course of chemotherapy treatment, but his body, exhausted and weakened by the earlier chemo, was unable to tolerate it and his kidneys started to fail. On 8 July, the family was advised to stop treatment and this they did. Anthony had only a few more months to live and, as his mum later observed, these were to become the most precious of his short life.

During the last phase of his life, despite his increasing fragility, Ant was able to enjoy several visits. On Friday, 21 June, I was pleased to accompany him to see the newly released film *Spiderman* at Brighton Marina. He had been looking forward to this film for some time. The advance publicity suggested that the portrayal of the adventures of his hero would be superbly done and perfectly in accordance with Ant's vision. The timing was appropriate to lift his spirits, after a long period of particular weakness and tragic news. His mum had been afraid that he would not be strong enough to visit the cinema, as by now he was increasingly tired and his breathing was becoming more laboured as his lungs weakened. At times, he was troubled by a distressing cough as he desperately struggled against the rapidly declining function of his lungs.

In the event, he was considered strong enough to visit the cinema in his wheelchair, as he had done to see *The Fellowship of The Ring* in January.

Anthony had hoped to be able to visit New York, largely, I think, to imagine himself with his great hero Spiderman, doing deeds of valour and swinging along the mighty canyons between the skyscrapers. Sadly, he was not strong enough to undertake such a demanding journey. In some ways, the film of *Spiderman* must have been appropriate compensation, for he was actually able to see his hero in action in all the vertiginous locations of which he had dreamed. As it was, the time of the release of this most apposite film for Ant was perfect. All those who loved him hoped that, at least for a few hours, it would take away some of the burden of distressing thoughts and fears that must have been pressing in upon him. I think our hopes were rewarded, for he was able to sit through the long film, clearly spellbound and without any discomfort and quite untroubled by his cough. Discussing the film afterwards, he told me that he was delighted by the fantasy, adventure and action he had seen depicted so well. It does seem that the film did afford him some bright diversion in his darkening days. Of course, the remarkable freedom, agility and sheer breathtaking adventure of *Spiderman* were exactly antithetical to Anthony's own experience of life at this time. As we shall see, this heroic freedom was to return in the remarkable circumstances of Ant's last moments.

On 4 July, Anthony started to be administered morphine to control the increasing pain in his lungs. This made him more sleepy and, now and then, uncharacteristically irritable. He also made increasingly frequent visits to the Royal Alex for long blood transfusions. These were to compensate for damage done to his bone marrow function, by the powerful chemo drug doxorubicin. His kidneys, too, never strong since his birth, had been damaged by the drug cisplatin and now they were failing.

On Sunday, 4 August, Anthony and his mum made an excursion in the Newhaven lifeboat as guests of the RNLI. Anthony sat securely on deck, muffled in a waterproof cape and sou'wester, while his mum made a video recording of the adventure. The weather was good and they sped through the swell, east, along the coast towards Beachy Head. During the trip, the lifeboat captain kindly explained, to a very attentive Ant, all that was happening. At one stage, much to the boy's delight, the men threw an unfortunate colleague overboard into the cold waters of the Channel, in order to demonstrate a rescue. They also showed the technique for a quick beaching, by charging through the breakers and up the shingle of Seaford Beach. This was a happy day for Ant, who returned home tired but full of good memories. The kindness and concern of these dedicated RNLI men, who gave so freely of their time, was much appreciated by all the family and will not be forgotten.

Having taken to the sea, Anthony's next experience, arranged by his mum, was in the skies over the Sussex coast. This was on Tuesday, 13 August, when Ant set out from Shoreham Airport in the aircraft used by the local radio station for reporting on traffic congestion. This time, there was no room for Gill, as the plane was only a small two-seater and Anthony had to take on the responsibility of using the video camera. The weather was again excellent as the little plane sped its way east over Brighton and along the coastline to Eastbourne. On the return trip, they made a special low pass over Ant's home at Peacehaven, all nicely captured by him on the video footage. This was Anthony's first flight, so it must have been a very exciting experience for him, heightened by the sense of nearness to the elements in the tiny craft as it bucked and banked in the onshore breeze. The deafening drone of the engine was partly decreased for Ant by his ear muffs, but the constant vibration transmitted by the frame of the light plane would certainly have added to the sense of adventure. Again, we were indebted to the kindness of these local people, who gave their time to enhance Anthony's remaining days. Each time I hear the little plane buzzing overhead, I am reminded of that happy day.

These excursions served as a precursor for another journey by plane. This time, a longer journey and a rather larger, less noisy plane. The holiday was, as things turned out, only a month before Ant's death. His mum and grandparents were able to take him for a week to Parc du Futuroscope, a theme park in western France, near Poitiers. They travelled out on Friday, 30 August, returning on Friday, 6 September. The flight was very difficult for Anthony, because of the cramped seating on the plane, but he was rewarded by the spectacular sound and light shows at Futuroscope, by the dinosaurs and by many other thrills. I still treasure the postcard he sent me and the little model dinosaur he so thoughtfully brought back for me. Again, the trip was recorded on video, to add to Gill's precious memories of her dear son.

On the weekend of Saturday, 28 September to Monday, 30 September, Gill and Anthony made what was to be his last excursion away from home. This was to be particularly enjoyable for Ant and it was the last time he was able to visit the annual games day arranged by Games Workshop at the NEC, Birmingham. This time, Anthony was too weak to go with his mates on the coach from Brighton. Instead, Gill drove him to Birmingham, where they stayed for two nights at Jury's Hotel, conveniently situated right next to the NEC. His friend Lewis met them at Birmingham. Again, Ant and Lewis were granted an early preview of the exciting new exhibits as Lewis carefully guided his friend's wheelchair around the show. Both lads enjoyed themselves and, once again, they spent a great deal of pocket money. This time, sadly, Anthony would be unable to complete most of the models that he had so happily carried home.

On Thursday, 3 October, I saw Anthony for the last time; my last glimpse of my beloved godson alive in this world. He was weak, but we were able to talk a little and to watch one of his favourite films, *Bicentennial Man.* It is the intriguing and touching story of a robot's 200-year journey to become a human being. Typical of Ant's interests, it explores the excitements, opportunities and costs of what it means to be human. I did not know, on that day, how appropriate this study of humanity would be within such a short time, to my thoughts, emotions and memories, as I mourned the loss of my dear godson. On Sunday, 6 October, I had my last precious words with him on the telephone. By now, his lungs were very congested and he could speak only with difficulty, so our conversation was brief. Anthony's distinctive and delightful voice and his happy mode of speech, so evocative of his presence, would be one of the greatest losses we had to bear. His chatter had filled the house with fun and purpose and now we would be brightened by it no more.

By Monday, 7 October, Anthony was desperately ill. He was unable to speak, because he was too weak and his lungs were blocked with tissue and fluid. He gasped for breath and he had to be given oxygen at frequent intervals. He lapsed in and out of consciousness.

As Anthony's mum sat with him through his last night (7/8 October 2002) he was very weak. At about 3.15 a.m. on Tuesday morning, to Gill's surprise, he became settled, conscious and was able to regain his normal breathing. Then, to her astonishment, he started to speak. (It is important, at this vital moment in Anthony's story, to bear in mind that the doctor, who arrived later in the morning, at once ruled out the possibility of Ant having been capable of speech; in his condition, it would be physically impossible, because his lungs would simply not have permitted it.) By his extraordinary determination and by the grace of God, we were able to glimpse a little of Anthony's transition from this world to the next. He found the strength to give his mum four distinct messages:

- He sounded excited and very happy, as though he had to drag himself away from what he was doing. 'I'm playing with my superheroes, Mum. They won't leave me alone. I've had to tell them to go away for a minute to let me talk to you.' His 'superheroes', of course, were the Marvel comic book heroes he adored, especially Spiderman and company.

- Then he said, 'Mum, I'm actually sitting, not in the bed where you think I am, but on the commode. I'm watching you from here and I can see you listening to me on the bed.' It seems that his spirit was now free to move, even though his body was incapable of rising from the bed. It is typical of Ant's humour, even at this moment, that he would choose the commode on which to perch, of all the chairs available in the room.

- He continued, 'Don't worry about me, Mum, I'm fine. A lovely lady has come to look after me. She's sitting on the chair next to me here. I don't know who she is, but she's very kind.' The mysterious and wonderful lady, though very present to Anthony, was invisible to Gill.

- He finished by saying, 'Mum, I can't hang on any longer. I can't do it any more.' Then Gill asked him to close his eyes and go to sleep. Having said goodbye to her, Ant took two more breaths and slipped gently into the next world. As Gill kissed him farewell, he was, she said, completely relaxed and at peace.

This was confirmed by the beautiful expression on his face, which I saw for myself, when I visited him for the last time in the funeral home that same evening. Those gentle features, so familiar to us, now beheld for the final time on this earth by those who loved him, radiated innocence, contentment and joy; surely the radiance of the Holy Spirit.

Anthony's medics feared that his final days and hours would be characterised by considerable pain. This was, of course, not the case. The fact that he died in peace and that he was able to speak at the point of death has confounded them and continues to do so. Francis, his nurse, who has made a special study of spirituality in terminally ill children, has told us that such experiences are not uncommon as children approach death. Jesus assures us of children's special distinction in God's eyes:

> See that you do not despise one of these
> little ones; for I tell you that in heaven their
> angels always behold the face of my Father
> who is in heaven.
> So it is not the will of my Father
> who is in heaven that one of these little ones
> should perish.
>
> (Matt. 18:10, 14.)

Anthony's amazing words as he was at the point of death have been a gift from God, of life-changing importance to Gill and to his family and friends. They were, and still are, a tremendous consolation to all who suffered with him and for him. We believe that we have been permitted to experience a glimpse of God's miraculous will (as promised by Christ), whereby suffering and death are transcended as the soul of an innocent child is carried by divine love into the glory of eternal life.

Jesus asks us to have faith in His promise; He who wept over the death of His friend Lazarus and who raised him to life (John 11:21–27). For, if our friend is the Lord, does not Lazarus represent every person who believes in Him? Christ's call of mercy will reach into the tomb for each of us, and raise us to new life with Him and with those we have loved and lost in this world.

As Anthony departed from this world on his amazing journey, it was diminished by his going. However, the arrival in heaven of such a gentle, humorous and brave little soul must surely be the cause for joyous celebration. The Book of Wisdom has words of reassurance for us:

The souls of the virtuous are in the hands of God,
no torment shall ever touch them.
In the eyes of the unwise they did appear to die,
their going looked like a disaster,
their leaving us like annihilation;
but they are at peace.
If they experienced punishment as men see it,
their hope was rich with immortality;
slight was their affliction, great will their blessings be.

(Wisdom 3:1–5.)

At his time of death, Anthony's age was 15 years and 9 months. The following chapters will consider the implications of what happened during those precious moments of Anthony's death.

Anthony's State of Mind

Before we examine the individual elements of what Anthony said as he approached his death, we should consider the evidence for his overall state of mind. It is worth remembering that as these remarkable words were spoken, Ant was talking to his mother, the person he loved above all others in the world and the person to whom he could talk most freely. She was the one who had never left his side during every moment of his arduous journey. In her, his love was reciprocated and she had his complete trust.

What strikes us first is the urgency of his message. There is a determination about it to explain to his beloved mum what was happening and to put her mind at ease. How was this possible? As he lay at the point of death he could not talk; his doctors confirmed that this would have been out of the question. His lungs were completely congested; he could scarcely draw breath for life, let alone form words. Besides, was he in any physical or mental state to think through what he may have wished to say? He was completely exhausted and *in extremis;* how he found the strength he needed we can but speculate.

Before he started to speak he had, to Gill's surprise, apparently roused from unconsciousness. If we suppose that, as seems to have been the case, Anthony was still fully in possession of his normal mental faculties, his determination to explain things to his mum and his wish to put her mind at rest are understandable. At his time of death, he seems to have been lucid and rational. He was, as we have seen, a young scientist; he was always keenly interested in observing what was going on. This was so right through his course of treatment and he frequently asked questions of his doctors and nurses. Similarly, he would not wish his mum to suffer at this terrible moment, if he could do something to help her. That he found a resolution to his determination at this late hour in his life, or that such a resolution was offered to him, is remarkable.

I am convinced from my knowledge of Anthony, and from the evidence of the circumstances we have before us, that he knew what an adventure he was going through. For him, these were new, amazing and exciting moments. But his love for his mum was his first concern, as was hers for him. She had brought him through his suffering thus far and now, in her final moment of agony, her arms still enfolded him and her loving face was before him still. Before he was carried away in the wonder of his journey, his imperative was to give her some assurance, some understanding and comfort. It is worthwhile reminding ourselves that all love comes from God and that God is love. It seems quite possible to me that our heavenly Father, in His compassion, raised Anthony from his affliction and 'gave him' to his mother in a very special way at the point of death. This is a mystery we cannot comprehend, but it can surely only have been done by the grace of God, so that the boy's wish to ease his mother's mind might be granted. How can we think less than this?

We are reminded of the story of the Widow of Nain in St Luke's Gospel, where we see Christ's compassion in similar circumstances:

11   Soon afterward he went to a city called Nain, and
     his disciples and a great crowd
12   went with him. As he drew near to the gate of the
     city, behold, a young man who had died was being
     carried out, the only son of his mother, and she was
     a widow; and a large crowd from
13   the city was with her. And when the Lord saw her,
     he had compassion on her and said
14   to her, 'Do not weep.' And he came and touched
     the bier, and the bearers stood still.
     And he said, 'Young man, I say to you,
15   arise.' And the dead young man sat up, and began
     to speak. And he gave him to his mother.

(Luke 7:11–15.)

The similarities are striking. Ant was a 'young man' and the only son of his mother. Gill may be regarded as a 'widow', her husband being no longer with her. Anthony 'rose', at least from the slumber of approaching death, and began to speak. God seemed to intervene and 'give' Anthony to his mother, if only for this short time. Of course, there are important differences. There were no great crowds. Anthony was not yet dead (as far as we can understand it), but at the point of death. The young man from Nain was presumably resurrected, until natural death overtook him at a later time. Nevertheless, the important lines for us are in verses 13, 14 and 15:

13   He had compassion on her.
14   And he said, 'Young man, I say to you, arise.'
15   And the dead young man sat up, and began to speak.
     And he gave him to his mother.

May we be allowed to consider that God's compassion was so invoked by the love between this dying young man (Anthony) and his mother, that He said, 'Young man, I say to you, arise.' In other words, He allowed Ant to describe the wonderful things that were happening to his mum, to give her some comfort and to say goodbye. The strength that was given to Ant to 'arise' and 'speak' certainly did not come from this world. His doctor was doubtful when Gill told him what had happened. He had insisted to her that it could not have been so, because it was physically impossible for him to have spoken. We are left to ponder over this amazing event and to dwell on its implications for our faith and for our lives.

Of course, there will be those, naturally more sceptical, who will say that none of this can possibly have happened. If the doctors said it could not happen, then it didn't. More likely, Anthony was in some morphine-induced state of euphoria (despite the fact that the general effect of the drug on him had been to induce lassitude and some irritability). Alternatively, could Gill have made it all up in her anguish or have convinced herself that she had heard words that were not actually there? We cannot definitely prove that this was not so. But the balance of probability is against it. We have the evidence of Ant's character and of Gill's character on our side:

- It is entirely in Anthony's character to want to do this, i.e. to say what was happening, to ease things for his mum and to say goodbye to her, whom he loved above all people.

- It is wholly believable that Ant's innocent soul, beloved by God, would cause Him to accede to the dying boy's loving concern for his mother.

- As with the widow of Nain, it is certain that the Lord's compassion was aroused by Gill's distress at the condition of her son.

- Gill is a practical, sensible and logical person, not given to deceit. She would not dream up any such story, let alone one containing such varied elements.

- Gill loved Anthony more than her own life. She would not have wished any untruth to be recorded about him, especially at this final moment in his life. She would have no reason or ulterior motive to concoct such a story. She carried no religious banner and did not wish to make any defence for God.

- Gill was as surprised by this turn of events as everyone else. She related the same story to all of Ant's family and friends and she faced the expected scepticism when she informed the medics. She did not offer, neither did she wish to, any explanation for the events, she just accepted them.

- Ant's doctors and nurses had already observed that, to their surprise, he was in no pain as he approached the end of his life. Cogent reason, perhaps, to accept a second surprise, i.e. that he actually spoke at the moment of his death.

The second quality that needs considering is the excitement Gill heard in Anthony's voice. How are we to understand the excitement conveyed in his voice and in his words, at what would be regarded as the most sombre moment in his life? Gill is quite clear about the excitement in her son's voice, because this added to the surprise of hearing him speak at all, at such a point in his illness. Not only could he speak, but he did so with enthusiastic fervour. He, who a moment before had been quite literally without breath, was now breathless with excitement.

The subject of his first words to his mother on this remarkable night (considered in the next chapter) do much to explain Anthony's excitement. But the fact that he was so excited at this point, and was able to be so, is so striking that we cannot avoid considering its implications. In common parlance, he was descending into death, into the sleep from which there is no awakening and into the termination of all consciousness. Anthony's experience as he approached death seems to invite quite a different insight. Hs faculties seem to have been heightened, his emotions charged and his consciousness full of the vibrant experience of joy. In short, in his spirit, he seems to have been rapidly awakening from the slumber of the sickness that had determined his life for so many months.

Some will claim that his experience was the result of elation, induced by the effect on the brain of morphine. This seems unlikely, as he had been taking the drug since July without any such effect and at his time of death his words were clear and balanced. If we discount the hallucinogenic influence of drugs, we still have to comprehend that what was happening to him appears to have been not just seen, but experienced by him as a living reality. We may invoke the chemical changes taking place in the brain at death by way of explanation of the not uncommon experiences of children, and others, as they leave this world. Whatever scientific explanation is called upon, wc still have the mystery that Anthony managed to relate his adventure using the power of his dysfunctional lungs. The evidence Anthony gives us in the strength of his own voice suggests an incredible paradox that as he entered into death he may have been, in his own experience, more alive than he had ever been.

Of course, it is part of the human condition that we cannot experience any other person's experience. You can experience me and I can experience you. But you cannot experience my experience of you and I cannot experience your experience of me. Thus arise many of the difficulties in human relationships. Consequently, we cannot be sure about Ant's own experience of what was happening. We have to take Gill's word for it. Neither can we experience her experience of being there. We are limited to experiencing her feelings as she tells us and by making our own judgements accordingly. This has always been the way of it throughout human history. People have to express in words what they have experienced inside their own minds, because we are all blind to one another's experiences. It is important to remember that we are no more disadvantaged with respect to Anthony than we would be with anyone else in this matter.

Thus, we can only speculate about Anthony's experiences on his own evidence, as we would with anyone else's. Of one thing we can be sure – what was going on in his mind had awoken him to an urgency and excitement that command our attention, especially when we remember that these were the last few moments of his life on earth.

Jesus makes an astonishing remark to His disciples in St Matthew's Gospel, which is certainly relevant to our remarkable line of thought:

> '...And as for the resurrection of the dead
> have you not read what was said to you by God,
> 'I am the God of Abraham,
> and the God of Isaac,
> and the God of Jacob'?
> He is not God of the dead,
> but of the living.'
> And when the crowd heard it,
> they were astonished at his teaching.
>
> (Matt. 22:31–33.)

Christ's use of the present tense indicates the eternal life that all the faithful have in Him. He is reminding us of what we so easily forget as we talk about our fear of pain and death, but never about His promise of eternal life. Although, in earthly terms, Abraham, Isaac and Jacob died long ago, God keeps them in life with Him always. He has no interest in dead people, but embraces all those He loves in everlasting life.

It is not surprising, of course, that the people were astounded at what Jesus said. Like most of us, they thought only in earthly terms. Jesus asks us to accept His promise that His heavenly Father does not want those He loves, especially His beloved children, dead. God asks His Son to suffer in the world, so that death may be defeated and those who love Him may enjoy eternal life. The First Letter of St John gives the same clear message:

> God is love, and he who abides in
> love abides in God, and God abides in him.
>
> (I John 4:16.)

If your heart is full of love, you already live in God and will continue to do so for eternity; for God also lives in you and will do so for evermore. If God lives in us by definition, we cannot die. God is love; if we live in love our souls are immortal.

It seems to me that only in Christ's remarkable promise do we find a cogent explanation of Anthony's experience of excitement and joy as he approached the portals of death. Anthony was an innocent child who, as we have seen, lived in love. Because he loved and was beloved, he was surely at one with God. In the virtue of childhood, he accepted God for what He is; the absolute and only condition for our existence. Thus, to use our Lord's terms, 'He believed in me'.

Our faith allows us to presume that although Ant's mortal body was to fade into dust on this earth, his immortal soul would be carried by the Son of God into eternity. At the moment of death, Jesus called him forth into new life as He called forth His friend Lazarus from the tomb and the young man of Nain to rise from the bier. Anthony's experience gives us a glimpse of these astounding truths and it leads us to live in joyful hope that one day, we shall be reunited with all those we love, body and soul, in God's new creation. Thus, we are strengthened to live in love and expectation.

The third quality we note about Anthony's state of mind is his complete lack of fear. Bearing in mind what we have considered above, this is, perhaps, not surprising. Fear is an emotion all too often associated with death. But, as we have seen, Ant's urgent concern to show his mum that all was well, combined with his excited happiness, impress upon us his absolute lack of fear. His whole state of mind appears to be one of complete security, freedom and confidence.

The conclusion we have drawn above as to the origin of the dying boy's excited demeanour, directs us to the source of his impregnable safety; he was secure in the love of God. Again, we remember our Lord's injunctions: 'Be not afraid' and, 'It is not the will of my Father in Heaven, that one of these little ones should perish'.

What need have we of fear, when instead we have such promises from the only human being who has ever lived in whom we can trust completely, the only person who has ever been fully human. Anthony was secure in this trust and his gentle young soul made the final stage of his journey, as he had endured the earlier phases, with complete bravery. This time, however, he was in ecstasy, not in suffering, as he demonstrates Christ's promise that love overcomes death. We need not fear death, for

Jesus has overwhelmed it in the fullness of His love and He has transformed it into a gift from God; a release from the suffering of the world and a gateway into a wonderful new dimension, where we shall be fully ourselves. It is, of course, also a gift of ourselves to God. We return to the Father who made us, into His loving arms, every one of us a prodigal son, sinner or saint. He loves us for what we are. He knows how and why we have failed and in His divine mercy He prepares for us a banquet at His heavenly table. All we need is faith in Christ, so that He knows us and welcomes us when the time comes for our own momentous journey.

In conclusion, we may summarise Anthony's state of mind at the time of his death in the following terms:

- Urgency in the need to get across his message to his mum in the little time he had available and in the nature and purpose of the content, which was to comfort his mother in her distress as much as he was able. His urgency was driven by his great love for his mum.

- Excitement at the amazing adventure opening before him as he was swept up into the love and wonder of his new life with the Creator of the universe, for whom all things are possible. For Anthony, the scientist, nothing could be more exciting than this. Of the wonders he has seen, we can but guess.

- Lack of fear. This little lad appears to defy death in his show of security, freedom and confidence. Such a lack of fear intimates his dependence on the all-embracing love of God, which enfolds him in unassailable bliss. Anthony's request to 'follow me' is validated by the unequivocal evidence of his state of mind as he enters into the next world.

> And when he had entered,
> he said to them, 'Why do you make
> a tumult and weep?
> The child is not dead but sleeping.'
> (Mark 5:39.)

Superhero

As Anthony awoke from his slumber, at the hour of his death, the first thing he told his mother was that he was having such fun:

'I'm playing with my superheroes, Mum. They won't leave me alone. I've had to tell them to go away for a minute to let me talk to you.'

Although his first message is superficially straightforward, it will repay detailed study. Each of the three sentences warrants careful consideration. Anthony begins by announcing what he is doing:

'I'm playing with my superheroes, Mum.'

First, we are struck by the fact that he seems to regard himself as being in another place, perhaps in another dimension or level of consciousness, or at least that he considers himself to have been elsewhere, until the moment before he returned to speak to his mum. He speaks in the present tense ('I'm playing'), suggesting that he is, or has recently been, active in mind, spirit and body. Gill, of course, until the moment of his awakening, has beheld his difficult slumber as he fitfully gasps for breath before her. Now, he awakes and, to her surprise, he tells her in the excited and urgent mood we have noticed in the last chapter that, in fact, he has been having enormous fun.

The most obvious interpretation of this is to assume that he has awoken from a dream. His body may be fading, but it seems that his mind is extremely active and has created for him a 'real' world in which he is able to join in play, no doubt energetically, with his superheroes. We all know how real dreams can be, but we also know that when we awaken, if we remember them, however vivid our memory, we recognise them to have been dreams; Anthony makes no such distinction. He is playing with his superheroes; to him, they are real and it is obviously his intention to return to them as soon as he has finished talking to his mum.

We may ask: why did he awaken from his dream at this point? How did he know that it was imperative to speak to his mother now, before he crossed the threshold of the next world? Anthony speaks as though he already lives in another place. Moreover, it is a place of such fun and delight that it seems to have been tailor-made for him. Could this joyful place manifest his new and heavenly home and has our Lord interrupted his play there to bring him to his mother for this special moment of farewell?

> Let not your hearts be troubled; believe
> in God, believe also in me. In my Father's
> house are many rooms; If it were not so,
> would I have told you that I go to prepare a
> place for you? And when I go and prepare a
> place for you, I will come again and will take
> you to myself, that where I am you may be also.
>
> (John 14:1–3.)

Surely Anthony's experience reaffirms our confidence in the wonderful promise that Jesus makes to those who love Him? The place prepared for my godson was, and is, a delight beyond belief for him and he is guarded by the everlasting presence of the Son of God.

We have considered the urgency and excitement of Anthony's state of mind as revealed by the tenor of his speech. This is confirmed by the subject of his first message, for he is playing with his 'superheroes'. His mum knew very well who these heroes were. For many years, Ant had collected books, videos, figures and electronic games and he had painted models and drawn the scenes that so vividly occupied his imagination. He had spent many happy hours entertained by the heroes of the *Marvel* comic world. Spiderman was the chief object of his fascination, but a whole range of little plastic superheroes was to be found on the shelves of his room. Anthony had continued painting his little figures during his illness, when he was strong enough to do so. He was very good at this, but only a few weeks before he died, not satisfied with his skill, he told me that he wished he could do better. I have no doubt that his favourite hobby, which gave him so much happiness, continues and that he is now the perfectionist he ever wished to be.

It is revealing to consider Ant's interest in the light of his personality, because this may help us to grasp the importance of his statement. As mentioned in the chapter on Sickness and Suffering, Anthony was still only a small boy at the time he was diagnosed with cancer. Though he was fourteen, he had not yet begun the growth spurt which characterises the teenage years. As we have also said earlier, he was quiet and considered in his manner, highly imaginative, intelligent and quick-witted. He had a few close and valued friends. He was not physically strong and he lacked the skills and the coordination to be a success at games. Moreover, he was not aggressive or competitive in any way. Thus, he was no sportsman; though, I think it is true to say that his friends saw him as a good sport, because of his ever-present sense of humour. Michael, his father, told me that as Anthony awaited the operation on his leg at Stanmore, he had asked Mr Briggs, his surgeon, if he would be able to play football when he recovered. On receiving the affirmative answer, Ant responded, 'Oh well, that'll be alright then, 'cos I never played it before!'

Despite his lack of prowess on the sports field, Anthony was never at a loss for what to do. He loved painting his Games Workshop figures and planning and playing battle strategies with the opposing armies of his schoolmates. They would spend all their pocket money on kits, models and equipment for their miniature war-games. Ant was also the avid reader of a series of fantasy stories, *The Animorphs*, by K. A. Applegate. These involved a group of young people who could metamorphose into animals, thereby assuming the powers and abilities of those creatures. Although not concerned with 'superheroes', the mythical fantasy and adventure in these books attracted Anthony and they gave an insight into his imagination. Any spare time he had, and he always found some by scooting through his homework as rapidly as possible, was devoted to one or other of his imaginary worlds. It seems as though Anthony compensated for his lack of ability in physical activities by using his creative imagination to the full.

The film *The fellowship of The Ring* similarly gripped Ant's imagination. The theme of the film is, of course, a heroic journey, during which a group of friends are beset by horrific and seemingly overwhelming dangers, but with mystical help, always arriving at exactly the right moment, they survive, The characters of *The Lord of The Rings* series were produced as models by Games Workshop, therefore making a link with Ant's hobby of model-making and painting.

We see that Anthony was very much a boy who lived in his imagination. In his mind, he created fantasy worlds where all things were possible. The psychiatrist Dr M. Scott Peck, writing in his book *The Road Less Travelled*, explains the development of the ego (the conscious self) through childhood. Between the ages of two and three, he says, children come to terms with the limits of their own power. They eventually come to appreciate their relative powerlessness in the world. But the dream of omnipotence, as he puts it, is so sweet that a child may escape for years into a realm of fantasy, where the possibility of its own omnipotence still exists. This, says Dr Peck, is exemplified by the world of Superman and Captain Marvel. He explains that as the child develops, these superheroes are given up, usually by the mid-teens.

Jung suggests that the myth of the hero is a personification of the deep longing of the unconscious, the soul, to be made real in the light of consciousness. The 'mythological images speak directly through the experience of external things'. Thus, the heroic dream is the yearning for the world to be 'made right', as we know in the depths of our hearts it should be right. In the world of fantasy there are many deep truths, which are recognised in the innocence of childhood. Anthony's heroes tell us much about the longing of his heart and he was never to lose this wonderful and intuitive awareness of the way the world should really be.

Anthony's death ensured that he never escaped from his superheroes. Perhaps his dreams were of superhuman abilities. In his fantasy world, he may have seen himself performing wonders and so becoming a renowned hero himself. Perhaps he just wanted to 'swing along' with Spiderman as an invaluable soulmate. Whatever his longing, it seems that by God's grace, his dreams were to be fulfilled as he entered into the kingdom of light. What are the characteristics of superheroes, like Spiderman? How do they fulfil the myth of omnipotence? They have great physical strength, plus superhuman physical abilities. In addition, of course, they have complete moral integrity and social responsibility. They are young, bold, energetic and 'clean-cut'. Often, though, they have a degree of mystery; usually, they are masked, so that the true identity of the heroes remains unknown to their admirers and foes alike. Anonymity is allied with a distinct lack of sexual involvement. There may be a hint of romanticism in the air, but the superheroes resist, keeping themselves devoted to their cause and eschewing relationships. This, of course, fits well with the developmental stage that precedes puberty, particularly with regard to boys.

Superheroes are, therefore, responsible citizens, who are always prepared to take effective action to protect the weak and the vulnerable and, in parallel, to overcome ruthless criminals, whose dastardly ambition is to prey upon society for their own devious purposes. It is notable that the criminals pitted against the likes of Spiderman are usually super-villains, anti-heroes, themselves possessed of extraordinary powers, almost the equal of their gallant adversaries. It is the quasi-religious, classic battle between good and evil; the epic struggle in which the heroes are given a bold run for their money and where the villains almost always have a bizarre attraction of their own. In these adventures, there are shades of *Paradise Lost* (where we have so much to admire in Satan); but, in the end, inevitably, paradise is regained when the heroes finally overwhelm their evil foes.

In the *Marvel* comic world, the 'ideal' that is being contested is the clean and wholesome, family-centred democracy of the American dream. A myth, itself, of course, and no less a myth than the wonder-man who protects it, or the bogeyman who threatens the established order. How often do we still build on such myths today, in the demons we see as threatening our society and in the usually political heroes who offer to protect us against them?

But the whole Captain Marvel construction is a simplified, exaggerated and idealised model of reality. For we do, indeed, live in a (much more complex) society, where goodness is threatened by evil and in which we frequently long for rescue by an omnipotent superhero. We, too, personify evil as though it always threatens us from without, not recognising the self-deception which lurks within our own hearts. In the stories of the superheroes, we have the satisfaction of always seeing good triumph in the end, unlike in the 'real' world, where good people frequently seem to suffer in their weakness and are often the victims of the powerful and the corrupt. These mythical stories fulfil a yearning in the heart of humankind for the victory of good over evil; a deep aching that has been reflected in human storytelling from the Greek heroes to the American cowboy and many tales of 'science fiction'.

It is probable that the *Marvel* superheroes attracted Anthony simply because of his gentle personality, combined with his innocent yearning for a world 'made right'. A whizz-kid on the computer, but a non-starter on the games field, did he, with his heroes, imagine himself capable of superhuman exploits? Did he see himself rescuing the needy, saving helpless victims, scaling the sides of skyscrapers and swinging through the man-made canyons of New York on urgent missions of liberation? It seems quite probable that this innocent fantasy might compensate for his much more routine everyday life at school, where he was quite content to take a modest role. Like Spiderman, he was self-effacing in his everyday life, only emerging as a wonder-worker under the cloak of anonymity; the mask of his make-believe. In his imagination, Anthony was living out a myth and as we consider his story we begin to glimpse the fundamental importance of the mythical aspect of Anthony's life. Jung claims profound value for a character trait we might too easily dismiss as juvenile fancy: 'The mythical character of a life is just what expresses its universal human validity'.

How remarkable that as Anthony was about to slip away from this world, we find him cherished by God, indulged by His boundless generosity. Did the God who is all knowing provide this gentle boy with his heart's desire as he became one among his superheroes? St Luke gives us a hint of the incredible bounteousness that awaits God's beloved children, as Jesus tells us,

> Judge not, and you will not be judged;
> Condemn not, and you will not be condemned;
> forgive and you will be forgiven;
> give, and it will be given to you;
> good measure, pressed down, shaken together,
> running over, will be put into your lap.
> For the measure you give will be the measure you get back.
>
> (Luke 6:37–38.)

These words give us the measure of God's generosity in the place He prepares for those He loves. They clearly indicate the path we must tread as we, too, seek to receive that love as we are united with Him and reunited in the loving embrace of those we have lost from this world.

In his dying words, 'They won't leave me alone', Anthony was not only able to play with his superheroes, to do what they could do, but he was the very centre of their attention. For they would not leave him alone or so he told his mum with joy; he had almost to push them away, to give himself the time to come and bid her farewell. The concentrated recognition his heroes seem to have been giving him suggests that he had become their superhero. For such a gentle and self-effacing lad, this experience must have been one of overwhelming affirmation. It is as though he was cradled in the palm of God's hand as his every wish was granted. In giving us this amazing glimpse into Ant's experience at that poignant moment, the grace of God allows us a confirming vision of His saving love. We are reminded of the bounteous welcome given to the prodigal son by his father (Luke 15:20–24). Although Anthony was a dutiful son and no prodigal, he seems to have enjoyed the bounty of God's love, just as described for the prodigal son. For as that son had suffered so, too, had Ant, though in his case through no fault of his own. Anthony is also the son who was dead and is alive again, who was lost and is found. The implications of this are profound. For we are certain that Anthony is alive in heaven, along with Abraham, Isaac, Jacob and all the countless throng of blessed souls who are received into God's kingdom. In the world, he was lost in his terrible illness and he came unto death. Now he is found and raised by the saving grace of Christ. Furthermore, he dines and makes merry at the heavenly banquet, together with all the saints in the light of God's face. Through his gentleness and innocence, he has transcended his suffering and receives his heavenly reward.

In his words, 'I've had to tell them to go away for a minute to let me talk to you', Anthony had to insist, almost joyously, in his new-found influence over his attentive heroes that they leave him for a moment, so that he can take care of his beloved mum. Obviously, he is reluctant to leave them, but now is the time he is called to say farewell to his mother. His love for her takes precedence over the fun he is having with his superheroes. At the same time, he heartens his mum and thus all of those who love him, by communicating the affirmation he is receiving from Spiderman and his allies. Formerly, Anthony had constructed this world in his mind and he was carried along in his own imagination. Now, to his surprise, no doubt, he finds his heroes coming to him in reality and welcoming him, as an honoured accomplice, into the centre of the action. He experiences them with all his senses. The heroes of his imagination have become real and the boy who has been bedridden for eighteen months finds himself with complete freedom and extraordinary powers. Anthony, it seems, is indulged by God's love as he is welcomed into his heavenly Father's house, just as Jesus has promised:

Truly, I say to you, unless you turn and
Become like children, you will never enter
the kingdom of heaven. Whoever humbles
himself like this child, he is the greatest in
the kingdom of heaven.

(Matt. 18:3–4.)

Anthony is both humble and innocent and he sets an example for us
as he enters the house of the Lord. Furthermore, he bids us 'follow
me' and we wait in joyful hope of the glorious day of reunion, when
every tear shall be wiped away. To take that path, we have to follow the
loving advice of our Saviour.

Having escaped from his heroes, Anthony is able to turn to his mum,
as God grants him the strength to speak to her. God 'gives him' to his
mother. This is a significant giving, the implication surely being that
Anthony's spirit will never be parted from his mother. As Ant takes
farewell of his dear mum in her distress, he is in effect saying to her 'Do
not weep. Be not afraid'. He is telling her that he has everything that
his heart could desire, not least her love, as he escapes from the anguish
of this world into the freedom of a new creation.

In his superheroes, Anthony had dreamed of extraordinary and
omnipotent power. Through his sickness, he was brought to the
complete weakness and emptiness of death. He had lost all power.
Then, in his utter poverty at his final moment, it seems that he was lifted
by Christ's mighty strength into the wonder of His resurrection; into the
everlasting power of God's saving love. The truth revealed in Anthony's
vision is that when we are powerless, we are open to receiving God's
power in the new life He gives us. As He saw Anthony, He sees each one
of us, His children, as a superhero, just as we are. He longs for our love,
He aches for us to turn our faces to Him; our Salvation.

A New Perspective

Having assured his mum of his immense happiness as he was indulged in boisterous adventures by his superheroes, Anthony moved on to explain to her his new-found freedom.

For eighteen months, he had been confined to his bed or, at best, his wheelchair. He could not walk unaided, because his left leg was painful and would not function properly. Also, as the months passed, his weakness and exhaustion inexorably increased. Moving him on any expedition out of the house could only be done when he was well enough and then it had to be planned carefully. Getting him to and from the car, and into and out of it, were major operations, at which Gill became expertly adept. She had to be, because of the many occasions on which he had to be taken to hospital for tests, transfusions and drugs. As his leg would hurt so badly when he had to be moved, Ant had complete trust only in his mum, his hospital nurses and his friend Lewis. He would let no one else move him.

It is fortunate that Anthony was not a sportsman, for although his confinement must have been extremely tedious and intolerable at times, he coped with it better than some boys would. Luckily, he was able to operate his computer. Like most young people, he was skilled at this and at playing computer games, many of which involved his superheroes. When he was relaxed enough, he would assemble his models and paint them. This gave him many hours of contented occupation. At less energetic times, especially towards the end, he enjoyed watching films. His favourites were those of his 'super heroine' *Buffy the Vampire Slayer* and of these he had a great collection. I remember reading of a mother in similar distressing circumstances, who would not allow her mortally ill son to watch his favourite films towards the end of his life, because she feared he would be 'wasting his time'. We had no such qualms about Ant; we knew he was deriving great benefit from his videos. They diverted his mind from his troubles and this was valuable even in the smallest way. They were also a source of brightness and of escape from the prison of his room into wonderful realms where anything could and did happen. The films he loved also provided Ant with many topics for the conversations he enjoyed – when he had enough energy for them.

Naturally, Anthony received many visitors during his illness, both from family and friends. We all became accustomed to seeing him, either in hospital or in the large hospital bed that had been installed in the living room of the family home. We had many happy talks. Anthony's sense of humour invariably prevailed and he loved quizzing his luckless visitors on the details of what he had told them, or what they had seen in his films, on previous visits. We became inured to seeing the reality he had to cope with every day; to his intravenous drips, to his liquid feeds through his gastrostomy tube and to the constant interruptions from nurses for check-ups, blood samples, pills and drinks. Sometimes, he was tired and just wanted to snooze. Then we would be privileged simply to be with him, to sit quietly and to ponder over all the happiness his life had brought.

With his visitors, Anthony was always calm, measured and matter-of-fact, though well aware of the seriousness of his condition. Unless very tired, he was easy to talk to and I often felt that, in his generosity, it was he who was doing his utmost to help us through our suffering as we beheld our beloved child in the grip of this terrible disease. He seemed to be aware of our feelings of helplessness and inadequacy and he was determined to do his best to ease our discomfort and to maintain our resolve to be brave. Only once did I weep in his presence. It was early on in his treatment, when he was suffering from appalling nausea from the chemotherapy and when he was as thin as a wraith because of his inability to eat or retain food. Bravely, he said, 'Now don't you cry, Ken, or I shall start. Then where shall we be?' We have remarked, in the chapter on Sickness and Suffering, on the rapidity of Anthony's maturation in his personality during his illness. His integrity and his intuitive perception of others were never to fail him.

The courage and dignity demonstrated by suffering children is frequently surprising and it often puts most adults to shame. Suffering or not, all human beings who have not reached adulthood, either in years or in development, are vulnerable, powerless and totally dependent. We see why Christ has so much love for children and why He holds them up to us as an example of those who are first in His kingdom. In their vulnerability and innocence, they are always near Him.

The routine visits to Anthony in the prison of his bed became so regular; a sad pleasure that was such a part of life, one felt they might go on forever. It was not to be, of course. Though, fortunately, when Ant found his freedom, the transition from this world to the next came suddenly and he was spared the serious pain that it was feared he might have to endure at the end.

At the hour of his death, the second revelation Anthony gave his mum was no less remarkable than the first. He seemed almost as surprised it was happening as she was to hear about it:

> 'Mum, I'm actually sitting, not in the bed where you think
> I am, but on the commode. I'm watching you from here
> and I can see you listening to me on the bed.'

He was at last experiencing the freedom he longed for, away from the confinement of his bed and from his broken body. He was not, he said, really on the bed with her, where she thought he was. He could clearly see her listening to him on the bed, but he did so from a new viewpoint. Because he was now sitting some yards from her, Anthony was seeing things from an entirely new perspective. The implications of this are as intriguing as they are remarkable. Consider the inferences we may draw from what Ant told his mum:

- Gill was sitting at the side of the bed listening to him. No doubt she was focusing on him intently as he lay there, ready to ease his breathing as much as possible by using the oxygen supply if necessary.

- Thus, his body was in the bed and he was talking there; his voice, a physical phenomenon, was coming from his physical body, as we should expect.

- However, Anthony's voice, which came from his body in the usual way, told her that his very self was elsewhere, not on the bed with his body, but sitting on the commode (some yards from the bed, but facing it).

- Furthermore, he was watching what was going on from his new vantage point, not from his bed where his eyes were obviously still located.

These four conclusions are somewhat disparate. We must, however, attempt to accommodate them in a coherent understanding of what may have been happening, in the subdued lighting of this ordinary sitting room in the early hours of that singular morning.

Seeing things from Gill's point of view, Anthony was firmly in the bed, as he had been for so many months. Admittedly, she was surprised by his sudden alertness, by his normal breathing and by the fact that he could speak to her. She had expected him to sleep fitfully during the night, as had been the case during the past few nights. He would waken her for oxygen, by using his alarm, if he had great difficulty with his breathing. His unexpected revival was, in itself, astonishing to her. And, of course, his doctors would later tell her that it should have been physically impossible for him to breathe normally or to talk. The condition of his lungs precluded any such activity.

The content of this part of his message was also surprising. As far as she was concerned, Anthony was on the bed before her; she held his hand to comfort him as any mother would. However, he claimed, from the bed, that he was not there, i.e. not where she saw his body. He was, he said, actually sitting on the commode, from where he could see her, and was not in the bed, where she could see him. Gill must have glanced, for a second, at the commode as he mentioned it. Naturally, she saw no one there. She may have allowed herself, even at such a sober moment, an instant of cheer in the familiar recognition of her son's humour in choosing the commode rather than one of the normal chairs.

This mother-and-son relationship was a very strong one, its strength reinforced by their mutual suffering. They understood and respected one another perfectly. Gill would not deny or disbelieve what her son had told her, particularly at such a moment as this, even though she lacked the credible evidence before her eyes. Similarly, Anthony would not have told his mother any untruth.

If we now consider Anthony's point of view, we come to the crux of the whole remarkable matter. For Ant's perspective had apparently changed quite literally; he was seeing things not from his body, but from outside of it. In fact, the whole point of this part of their brief, final conversation that night, is that he wanted to tell her of his amazing change of vision. He could see his mother listening to him as he was talking to her, but he saw his mum and himself from a new point of view, some distance away. It was as though she was talking to his empty shell. The reality of the situation must have been, if anything, even more surprising for Ant than for Gill. She had only to consider what he had told her (though incredible) and no other supporting evidence, apart from her absolute trust in what he had said. He, however, could clearly see his own body a few yards away from him. He seems to have accepted this with equanimity. He was seeing things in a new light.

We have no alternative but to accept Gill's account of things for, as we have said earlier, there would be absolutely no point in her fabricating such a remarkable story. In the circumstances, the only possible conclusion I believe we can come to is that Anthony's spirit was now outside of his body, separated from it in some way. Why or how this happened is a mystery. It is clear, though, that he wanted his mother to know this incredible change in the very nature of his being. A surprising change it may be, but he does not seem to have been at all disturbed by it. He was not frightened, but delighted to tell his mum of his new-found freedom.

If we assume that Anthony's spirit had separated from his body in some way, the logical question to ask is was he at this stage actually dead? It is commonly supposed that the soul or spirit of a person, the very core of his or her being, separates from the body at the point of death. The body, being material and corruptible, returns to the earth as dust; the spirit, being immortal, returns to God from whom it came. When he said these words, however, the evidence is that Anthony was not yet dead. The words themselves presumably came from his living body. He was still breathing in order to form those words; though, as we know, this was a minor miracle in itself. Admittedly, he was very close to death, because he would only breathe for another minute or two, at the most. Nevertheless, it seems that Anthony's spirit found freedom from his exhausted body at some stage before the physical processes of life ceased.

For Anthony, this must have been remarkable, and for the young scientist that he was, exciting and intriguing. His eyes had been opened to a new vision of reality and his soul was joyously free, waiting for the Lord in expectation of the wonders to come:

> I wait for the Lord, my soul waits,
> and in his word I hope;
> my soul waits for the Lord
> more than the watchman for the morning,
> more than the watchman for the morning.
>
> (Psalm 130:5–6.)

It is typical of him that he wished to tell his beloved mum what was happening to him. For her, it was an incredible comfort to know from her son that he had now found freedom at last, from all the pain and suffering that he had so long endured in his earthly body. That his spirit was alive, well and happy was a gift to Gill of immense value. She was brought some consolation for the tribulation they had both experienced for so long. She knew for certain that she was to lose the beloved physical presence of her son, but at the same time she sensed that he would still be with her. Their love would survive his death. Moreover, Anthony had found the strength to give her this consolation at the moment of his death; an act of devotion and love and one of the most poignant moments in the story of Anthony's amazing journey.

Where did Ant's remarkable strength at his weakest moment come from? I am sure that this whole incredible event arose out of love, through love and for love. We know that God is love. The only possible understanding we can have is that God, in His gracious love, reaffirmed the eternal bond between this suffering mother and her son. Christ transformed their suffering into a message of hope for Gill and thus for all who love Anthony. The hopelessness, meaninglessness and pain caused by this innocent boy's terrible suffering reveals an immense poverty; an absolute necessity for God. Where human love and suffering coexist in this way, as they so often do in our damaged world, it seems that God, in His boundless compassion, may send His Son to those who suffer. Christ shows Himself to them in His glory and brings His healing and peace. As in the story of the Widow of Nain, we must believe that Jesus 'gave' the dying Anthony to his mother. She knows that her son lives and that she has his love and that he has hers for eternity. They will never be separated in spirit and one day they will be reunited, body and spirit in God's new creation. (This was to be confirmed in Anthony's third revelation to his mum, discussed in the next chapter.)

The glimpse Anthony gives us of an existence beyond death is compelling and comforting. His experience seems to confirm the possibility of some sort of separation of spirit and body at or near death, i.e. as we approach our Creator. Holy men and women, who practise contemplative prayer, also sense a separation of spirit and body as they draw near to God in the profound depth of their prayer. They then seem to live in the spirit with God and to lose all sense of their bodies. They come to see that we are, in reality, spiritual beings and temples of the Holy Spirit. God dwells within our hearts. Monks and nuns, who are contemplatives, speak of the delightfulness of the separation of body and spirit. They feel, as did Anthony, that as the spirit slips away from the body, this is perfectly acceptable. It seems to them to be no great change and it is not frightening in any way. Quite the reverse, for the fear of death is vanquished when we know what it is like for the body and the spirit to be separate.

Rumi, the thirteenth-century Persian mystic, wrote: 'When the bodily medium is removed, he who is disembodied perceives without any screen, like Moses, the light of the Moon shining from his own bosom.' In other words, in the spirit, we are able to stand before God, just as Moses did, and like him, we return from God, effulgent with the uncreated light of His glory. We can scarcely imagine how marvellous this will be for Anthony; the curious young scientist will have all his questions answered as he beholds wonders beyond our comprehension. Even more incredibly, his dreams will be fulfilled as he discovers that his own powers and abilities exceed those of his 'superheroes'. We, who love him and remain in the world, know how much he deserves every exciting moment of his new life.

Because the spiritual part of a human being is of God, it is of love. To grow spiritually we have to grow in love. We are assisted in this by God's many gifts of grace, most notably the gift of His love, the Holy Spirit, who is able to dwell within us as guide and counsellor. As we increase in love, we grow nearer to God, nearer to the goal of life's journey. Anthony has shown us that a person who is spiritually mature has died to his or her own self and that such a person follows in the footsteps of Jesus. Anthony's innocent and loving spirit was certainly with God already as his body approached death. He knew the momentous nature of what he was saying when he asked us to follow him, for he already had a clear vision of his brilliant journey's end. Anthony's courage inspires us to follow, in certain hope, the pathway through our own suffering lives.

Behold, Your Mother

We now come to the most mysterious and wonderful part of Anthony's message:

> 'Don't worry about me, mum, I'm fine. A lovely lady has come to look after me. She's sitting on the chair next to me here. I don't know who she is, but she's very kind.'

Each of these four sentences will benefit from detailed consideration. His first words here again seek to reassure his mother:

> 'Don't worry about me, mum, I'm fine.'

The sentence echoes Jesus' 'Be not afraid', repeated so many times to His disciples. Anthony again shows his concern for his mum as he endeavours to give her strength in her moment of extreme distress. We remember that Mary, the mother of Jesus, stood at the foot of the Cross, where she watched the agony and death of her Son. Gill, like so many suffering parents, is brought to the foot of the Cross. Here, she watches her own son as he faces death. As with Mary she, who carried him in her womb, nurtured him, brought him into the world, cared for him, taught him and loved him with all her strength, watches her son suffer and depart. She, full of tenderness and love, overwhelmed with sadness, is powerless and helpless. By the power and grace of God, Anthony is given the strength, at the moment of his death, to follow our Lord's example in giving comfort to his mother in her distress:

> But standing by the cross of Jesus were his mother
> and his mother's sister, Mary the wife of Clopas
> and Mary Magdalene. When Jesus saw his Mother,

and the disciple whom he loved standing near,
he said to his mother,'Woman, behold, your son!
Then he said to the disciple, 'Behold, your mother!'
And from that hour the disciple took her to his own home.

(John 19:25–27.)

Jesus said to Mary from the Cross, 'Woman, behold, your son,' referring her to John, His beloved disciple, who stood with Mary and the other women at the foot of the Cross. Jesus was passing His mother into John's care. We might imagine our Lord using the same words to Gill as she waited at the foot of Anthony's bed: 'Behold, your son.' As we have seen in the chapter on Anthony's State of Mind, God seems to 'give' Anthony to his mother for this short time. To Anthony, as to John, the words would have been: 'Behold, your mother'. It allowed a final (and divine) strengthening in this world of the bond between them and it granted a parting consolation to Gill, as only her beloved son could give it. She needed no other and, indeed, no one else can possibly grant her any such comfort, however much they may wish to. Only Gill had this experience of her son at such a profound moment and no one can take it from her, just as she will never lose the joyous memories she carries of her life with Anthony.

Why was there a need for reassurance at this point in Anthony's words? Could it be because he was to lead on to his most momentous announcement? Perhaps Ant's greatest distress in his illness had been to witness his mother's suffering, to behold her increasing exhaustion, day after day, as she drained herself of energy to provide for all of his many needs. He depended on her completely and he loved her above all others. He now had something of supreme importance to tell her; it would be a surprise and the last thing he wanted to do was to shock her. So he prepared her. What he was saying, in effect, was: you can relax, mum, don't be afraid for me, everything will be alright, because I'm being taken care of exactly as you take care of me.

Now, at last, we come to the very centre of his message, the almost inexpressible core of what he has to tell his mum during his final moments in her arms; of the incredible vision he beholds, that she cannot see. For they are not alone in the room. In the silent gloom of this ordinary sitting room, in the depth of the night, they are joined by a third person, a lady of incomparable beauty:

'A lovely lady has come to look after me.'

Why did he say she was lovely? Did he simply mean that she had a lovely face? Or was he suggesting she was a lovely person? If the former, we assume that he had certainly had the time and the opportunity to get a reasonable look at her and thus to appreciate the beauty of her appearance. If the latter, then more familiarity is implied. By using the term 'a lovely person', we usually invoke such qualities of personality as delightful, gentle, pleasant, happy and considerate. A 'lovely person' is certainly one we should be pleased to be with, because he or she is not only well-disposed towards others, but is a person who also puts others' concerns first. We might well put our trust in a 'lovely person'; we could rely on that person and we would be guided by him or her. To appreciate that persons are 'lovely' in this fuller sense means either that we know them quite well, and we have had the time and experience of them sufficient to trust them, or that in some remarkable way they have so quickly been able to impress us with their integrity that we are completely convinced. With Anthony's experience of the 'lovely lady', it seems that the second of these must have been the case, for we have no evidence that he knew the lady before.

Anthony does not describe the lady's appearance. He just tells us that she was 'lovely'. It seems fairly certain that he was impressed by her beauty. I do not think he would have used the all-embracing term 'lovely' otherwise. She was beautiful and he was struck by her beauty, but the beauty of her appearance was, to him, only the outward and visible sign of a deeper and more fundamental beauty; a beauty of personality, of humanity, so captivating and engaging that he was rapt, enfolded in her warmth and love, from the moment he saw her. How long, in temporal terms, she had been present to him is, in a sense, irrelevant, because the wonderful and inviting aura of trust she radiated was so overwhelming that he just knew it as soon as he saw her.

Whatever the truth about how he came to this understanding of his mysterious lady, it is certain from his brief words that Anthony was greatly impressed. He must have been totally convinced of her integrity and of her love for him. The lady was obviously present to Anthony and for Anthony. He need not have told his mum about her, but he wanted to do so (as we have said above), to reassure her not to be worried, because he was completely convinced of the lady's incredible worth as a person. He had given her the seal of his approval and he knew this would be an absolute confirmation for his mum. He was not going to be abandoned. The tender care that the woman he loved above all had provided without stint for so long would continue to be there for him as he moved into the ultimate adventure. Whoever this lady was, she would love him with his mum's love. He meant no less than this and his mother was convinced of it.

As to the fact that the 'lady had come', we do not know when she had arrived or where from. We know that Anthony believed her to be in the room, but we have no clue as to how she got there. Anthony does not tell us and, in any case, he may not have known. But there are some insights we can draw from these words. The very fact that she had come (from somewhere), implies that she had not been there earlier. At some stage, he had become conscious of her and he had quickly been able to appreciate her qualities. The fact that she had arrived for him must have made him aware, at this transforming moment, that he would not be alone after he had taken his earthly farewell of his mum. The lady would carry on the flow of his mum's enduring love into his new life; she had easily been able to convince him of that. The fact that she had come for him was the significant point, not where she may have come from. We may return to the latter question when we come to consider the lady's possible identity.

She had come to be with Anthony. Furthermore, he tells us specifically that she 'has come to look after me'. He knew this and was in absolutely no doubt about it. He made sure he told his mum, because this was the essential part in her reassurance. His certainty on this point presents us with a most intriguing question: how did he know that she had come to look after him? There are three possibilities:

- She must have spoken to him and told him this.

- Someone else must have done so.

- His certainty on the point must have been communicated to him by the lady (or by someone else) in some unspoken way.

If we assume that she spoke to him, we are faced with some fascinating potentialities. What, for example, was her voice like? Was it a contributory part of her loveliness? Even more importantly, what did she say? She may have told him more than that she had come to look after him. If she had spoken to him or, even more significantly, with him, we may guess that she was probably concerned enough to comfort him. Whatever words she may have used, she undoubtedly put him at his ease and won his confidence, thus confirming what we have deduced of her nature. Anthony would almost certainly have wanted to know where she had come from, who she was and what the next stage of his adventure was likely to be. Perhaps some of these things he already knew but, at this stage, anyway, he did not know who she was. This indicates that if they had spoken it may, thus far, have been only briefly. It would also suggest that the trust he had placed in her was more the result of some direct and mysterious communication of love from this wonderful lady to Anthony, rather than the outcome of any familiarity built up over a period of time. We may probably conclude that he had not known her for long, but that she already had his complete confidence and that he was certain that the whole purpose of her being there was to take care of him.

It seems unlikely that Anthony's information (and therefore his understanding of the situation) came from some other person or surely he would have been struck by the fact and mentioned it? Our conviction must be that Ant's reassurance came, either directly or indirectly, from 'the lady' herself.

The understanding we have arrived at may allow us to return briefly to the initial sentence of reassurance, which preceded Anthony's revelation about the lovely lady. How could he have been so sure he was 'fine'? There was no fear in what he was saying, despite the fact that he had before him a lovely and unknown lady, who had mysteriously arrived 'from nowhere', a lady whom he appeared to understand that his mum could not see. Surely this is corroboration that she had already spoken to him or comforted him in some way? Had she already told him what was happening? We do not know, but it is quite certain that she had managed to reassure him that all was well at this potentially frightening time for him. Anthony's concern was to pass on this reassurance to his mum.

> When the Lord has given you
> the bread of suffering and the water of distress,
> he who is your teacher will hide no longer,
> and you will see your teacher
> with your own eyes.
> Whether you turn to right or left,
> your ears will hear these words behind you,
> 'This is the way, follow it.'
>
> (Is. 30:20–21.)

Anthony had certainly been given 'the bread of suffering and the water of distress'. Just as Isaiah had promised, his teacher came to him. As it turned out, Anthony's teacher was a lady rather than the man indicated in Isaiah's prophecy. But it is likely that Jesus, the teacher of us all, sent the lovely lady to Ant. Her purpose was to show him the way to his eternal home. She was 'the Hodegetria', the One Who Points the Way. From Isaiah we learn that, in all probability, she did speak to Anthony; indeed, he could scarcely avoid the words of his delightful but importunate companion. In contrast to what he has just told us, Anthony's next revelation about the lady, though surprising, is quite factual and straightforward:

'She's sitting on the chair next to me here.'

We are at once struck by the domestic normality of the remark. But things are far from normal. A mysterious lady, who has appeared out of nowhere, with whom he is already completely comfortable and whom his mum cannot see, settles herself down in the familiar chair next to him, in the ordinary surroundings of this suburban sitting room, in the dead of night. We add to the singularity when we remember that the Anthony the lady is sitting with is his disembodied spirit, not his physical presence, which remains on the bed with Gill. The whole scene is almost an absurd ambiguity, a paradox. Were not the circumstances so serious, we might be tempted to dismiss the entire situation as an inconsistent enigma, not worthy of further consideration. We know otherwise, of course, when we take into account the context of Anthony's experience on this, his final night on earth.

Anthony's remark, though seemingly innocuous, allows us to ask some more questions about what was taking place:

- Why did he say where the lady was?

- Why was she sitting next to Anthony?

- Why was she sitting at all?

These questions, though simple, are not worthless, because it is only by persisting with consideration of the detail that we may shed a little light on the remarkable events that were taking place and move towards an understanding, or an acceptance, of what this brave boy was experiencing at the moment of his death.

Anthony told his mother exactly where the lady was. She was sitting on a chair next to the commode already occupied by his own disembodied self. Why was he concerned to let his mum know where the lady was? Because, by sitting next to Anthony, it was quite clear that she had come to be with him, to grant him the comfort of her presence. Just as we, his loved ones, had visited his bedside at hospital and at home on many occasions during his illness, in order simply to be with him. Few words were needed on those loving visits. We were just with him and there for him, the child we loved.

As Ant prepared to fade from this world, it was as though the lovely lady was taking on this role, a loving presence we could no longer provide. Furthermore, she, a loving lady, who had already gained his complete trust, had arrived, it seems, to continue into eternity the unique and essential love of his mum. For how can a child manage without his mother's love? Anthony's first and his only wish, as he passed into the life to come, would surely be to have his mother's love with him. It cannot have been otherwise. I believe that wish granted, for He who loves children and seeks always to protect them will not neglect the dying wish of an innocent child. Anthony was moving from the suffering of the world we have broken, into the kingdom of heaven, where God's will is done.

As the lovely lady sat on the chair next to Anthony, we have no certainty about what passed between them, except for one thing; the most important gift one human being can give another – love. She chose her place next to him to be with him and to be at one with him. The choice of her place at his side was one of divine affirmation.

Why was she sitting? Why did she not simply enter the room and stand at his side? When someone comes and sits with us, we know that they wish to be with us for more than a moment. Indeed, we have all experienced that occasion when we have asked a visitor or visitors we love to sit near to us, to stay with us, to remain for more than a brief call. We would like to enjoy their company and we would hope that they should want to be with us. And when we go and sit with a friend, especially if he or she is unwell, we know that we are, in fact, waiting with them. We are giving them our time, waiting there with them, as our friendship and love require. We wait with them, because we want to be with them on life's journey.

As the lady sat next to Anthony, she was waiting with him in another sense, too. She waited while he made his farewells to his mum and so to all those he loved. By sitting with him, she behaved as any kindly human being would if she were waiting for him to complete a task he had to do.

Was she also waiting for something else? Would they be going somewhere together? Had she come to take him, to guide him on his journey? We are reminded of those wonderful icons of Mary, the Hodegetria, the One Who Points the Way: Mary, the loving and tender Mother, the Mother of God and therefore of all mankind. She points the way to our ultimate destiny, to her own beloved Son, to our Redeemer and our salvation.

Anthony concludes his message about the lovely lady by saying, 'I don't know who she is, but she's very kind.'

His conclusion is abrupt and almost startling, but again it will reward close study. For of these few enigmatic words we can ask several questions that may increase our understanding of this most crucial step in Anthony's momentous journey.

Why did he not know who the lady was? Simply because he had not seen her before? Probably, but we can still demand more of these meagre words, if we bear in mind what has already been said about the mysterious lady.

We are fairly certain that Anthony had seen her face clearly, for he had described her as 'lovely'. So he had taken note of her features and appreciated her beauty, but he did not recognise her as anyone he knew. Either she was someone he did know and her appearance had changed in some way so that he failed to recognise her or he had never seen her before. If the former, we are reminded of the occasion, following Jesus' resurrection, when Mary Magdalene completely failed to recognise Him in the garden, near the tomb:

> She turned round and saw Jesus standing there,
> but she did not know that it was Jesus.
>
> (John 20:14.)

Similarly, on the road to Emmaus, two of Christ's disciples do not know Him when He joins them on the road. They do not recognise Him until they eat supper with Him that evening:

> When he was at table with them, he took the
> Bread and blessed and broke it, and gave it
> to them. And their eyes were opened and
> they recognised him.
>
> (Luke 24:30–31.)

These failures to identify Jesus, in both cases a close and much loved friend, seem strange, but at the threshold of heaven we are contemplating mysteries beyond our comprehension. Anthony's lovely lady certainly appeared to know him well and as we have said, she obviously came to be with him and was full of tender care for him. So we are left with the inevitable conclusion that she knew him, but he did not know her. This will be important when we come to consider the origin of the mysterious lady.

How did Anthony know, with such confidence, that she was so very kind? We can invoke the same line of reasoning we used when contemplating how he knew, for a certainty, that she had come to look after him. She must have communicated with him either verbally or non-verbally, most probably both. It is worth remembering that we discern people's attitudes towards us both by what they say and how they say it. Kindness can be conveyed in the tenor of the voice; we may read attitude from facial expression, bodily expression and posture and also from gestures. To a child, a loving woman would naturally convey kindness by a kiss, a hug, perhaps, and a warm holding of the hand. We cannot know if any of this happened, but we can suppose that some of it, at least, must have done, for Anthony was certain in his mind of the lady's kindness. To what effect was this kindness? To a child in Anthony's ultimate moment of need it was essential; the prevenient grace of the love to come. It would banish all fear and it would open the gates to the glorious new world of safety, tenderness, compassion and magnanimity. We remember, here, another group of icons: those of Mary the Eleousa, the Mother of Loving Kindness. In these beautiful paintings, the love expressed between Mary and her Son is of exquisite tenderness. Love overwhelms the beholder and draws us into the eternal relationship. This, of course, is exactly what was happening to Anthony in the presence of this beautiful, incomparable lady. He was being drawn into heaven; her compelling love was utterly irresistible.

Finally, we approach an intriguing question about Anthony's mysterious lady. Who could she have been? We know many of her characteristics: she was not frightening, she was beautiful, she had come to take care of him, she was near him and she appeared to be waiting for him, he did not recognise her and she was very kind. Unfortunately, although she was a paragon of virtue, she is still not clearly identified for us. We can believe that in the wonder of her person and in the role of her mission she may have been Mary herself. But she could have been an angel, a deceased relative or, less likely, a completely unknown person. We cannot know for certain, but we can draw out some threads from our own beliefs, from scripture, from the Church and its prayer and perhaps from the apparition of Mary at Fatima, eighty-five years before Anthony's death. Any threads, which correspond, which support one another, are more likely to point towards the truth. This is called the 'coherence theory of truth', suggesting that the available evidence, however sparse, at least fits together to produce a coherent whole. It is theory, not fact, so at best we can only hope for an indication of the lady's possible identity, while allowing for individual preferences of interpretation and for scepticism.

It is worth returning to the events at Fatima in Portugal, which were first mentioned in the chapter on Sickness and Suffering, in connection with Anthony's 'angel'. In May 1917, some time after they had seen the angel, these same children had a vision of Mary. For our purposes, we may discard the peripheral detail and concentrate on the appearance of Mary in the Fatima vision. The children said that there was a flash of lightning, followed by a dazzling and wonderful apparition. They described a circle of light with a beautiful lady standing in its centre. Her dress was as white as snow and a white veil covered her head and shoulders. She held her hands together, as if in prayer. Her face was of ineffable beauty and it shone in the light of a brilliant halo. The 'lady', for that is what they called her, spoke to them with motherly kindness. The beautiful lady appeared to the children several times and it was not until one of her later visits that she identified herself as Our Lady of the Rosary.

We noted how Anthony's 'angel' was very similar to the angel seen by the children at Fatima. With respect to the 'lovely lady', the similarity of the experience seems equally striking. Immediately after Anthony's death, I phoned my brother to tell him of the tragic news and the singular circumstances of the hour of Ant's death. When I had related his words about the mysterious lady, my brother was at once struck by the remarkable concordance between the boy's words and those of the children at Fatima. The three outstanding points of correlation are:

- Both the children and Anthony found the lady they saw extremely beautiful or lovely.

- At both events, they experienced the lady as being incredibly kind.

- In both circumstances, they did not know (initially in the case of Fatima) who the lady was.

I had not then read the details about Fatima and so did not make the connection. But my brother recognised the link as soon as I told him of Anthony's experience.

This correlation certainly puts the identification of Anthony's lady as Mary in a positive light. At first, the Fatima children did not recognise their lady as Mary, but she subsequently revealed her identity. Her similarity with Anthony's lady is without doubt and the lady of his vision certainly has all the remarkable attributes we should expect of the Mother of Jesus. Is it too much to suppose that Anthony could have beheld Mary as he lay at life's end in that ordinary and unassuming house? We have seen how Mary is regarded as the 'Hodegetria', the One Who Points the Way. The wonderful, kind and beautiful woman who came to wait with Ant was certainly there to guide him on the most important stage of his journey. And she was no ordinary guide; she captivated his heart and she put his mind at rest, with a love akin to his own mother's love. In this, she shows also the characteristics of the 'Eleousa', the Mother of Loving Kindness, the other iconic view of Mary that we have mentioned.

We wrote of Gill's identification with Mary, in the extremity of her suffering, as she waited with loving tenderness for the death of her own son, treasuring, as she must have done, each precious moment. The scriptures tell us that Mary, a humble peasant girl, was chosen by God as perfection among women, to bring His own Son into human flesh. Her simple assent to the Angel Gabriel ensured that she is the personification of love, humility and kindness for eternity.

Who but Mary, who had waited at the foot of the Cross for her Son's agony to be over, could be chosen by God to bring His beloved children to Him at the hour of their death? An angel could not be chosen for such a profound task; it must be the human being, who has suffered in the world the ultimate bereavement. One of the most ancient prayers of the Roman Catholic Church is the Hail Mary (the prayer of the Rosary):

> Hail Mary, full of grace, the Lord is with thee.
> Blessed art thou among women,
> and blessed is the fruit of thy womb, Jesus.
> Holy Mary, mother of God,
> pray for us sinners now
> and at the hour of our death. Amen.

For centuries, the Church has acknowledged that it will be Mary who intercedes for us with God at the hour of our death. She will pray for us now and then, when these two moments will become one as we pass into eternity. We beg for her loving intercession, through her Son, for our life now and for our death, which leads to everlasting life. In effect, we ask her to guide us on our journey to her Son, who is the Lord of time and space and the Lord of eternity. Mary lives with us as we face death and we move with her along the journey from the present, through the awful barrier of death. Her love and compassion carry us beyond the human tragedy of death, to the victory of love over death gained for us by her Son.

Some will believe that it is a loving relative, already garnered unto God, who comes to receive the soul of the departed at the moment of his or her death. I would not wish to deny such a belief. The fact that Anthony did not recognise his lovely lady does not mean that she was not some long since dead relative he had never met or that he was too young to remember. That she was lovely, kind and totally concerned for him would be explicable, both in terms of her relationship to him and because she had presumably come from heaven to receive him. She would, in any case, be doing Mary's work for her, bringing the love of the Mother of all mankind to a needy soul at the hour of death. She would be imbued with the spirit of Mary to such an extent that she would, in a sense, be at one with Mary – indistinguishable in love, mercy and purpose.

Who is Mary but the loving mother of us all? The significance of Mary's attention at the end of our lives is precisely because Mary's love is a mother's love: forgiving, accepting, tender and merciful. To the extent that a mother loves her child, she becomes at one with Mary. That is why, in the end, I believe Anthony was so content, so secure, because he was still receiving his own mother's love from this wonderful lady, whatever identity we give her. In her grace and kindness she embodied all he had ever wanted and all he had received in abundance in this earthly world from his mum. As we have said, it is scarcely likely that God, who in His bounteous love provides 'superheroes' for Anthony's delight, would deny the little lad's most earnest request for his beloved mum to be with him. She was with him, she is with him and she always will be, because it is love that has vanquished death. 'Behold, your mother' might well be the words our Lord whispered in Anthony's ear as, entering into heaven, the recognition of the lovely lady's identity began to dawn on him at last. The atonement for his suffering would then be complete. God's promise to us is quite clear:

> As one whom his mother comforts,
> so I will comfort you.
>
> (Is. 66:13.)

Why the slow dawning of such recognition? We cannot understand this mystery but, as mentioned earlier, when the resurrected Christ first appeared, there were occasions in which those who loved Him failed to know who He was.

To those who would object to the temporal anomaly, by suggesting that it would be impossible for Gill, who remains in this world, to be with Anthony in any sense, if he is now in heaven, we can begin to perceive an answer. The kingdom of heaven is not bound by constraints of time and space. It was, is and ever shall be. It is eternal. Love is what transcends the boundary between the temporal and the eternal. That love between mother and son, established on earth, was already in the eternal realm; an example of how the kingdom of heaven breaks into our world now. Gill's love will be there for Anthony always, as will his love for her. It is a spiritual truth and, of course, it is impossible to wrap up such profound mysteries in words. In the end, we have the security of God's rhetorical question to Abraham:

> Is anything too hard for the Lord?
>
> (Gen. 18:14.)

There is one more connection with Mary we can draw from the months of Ant's illness. That is the holy water from Lourdes he was so kindly given by his teacher Kit Wood. Lourdes, like Fatima, is the site of an apparition of Mary (in 1858). It is perhaps the most renowned Marian shrine and a centre of pilgrimage for sick people (especially children) from all over the world. Many miracles are recorded from the healing waters at Lourdes and much solace and comfort is granted to the many more who are not healed. Anthony certainly had much faith in his little bottle of holy water and he dutifully applied a small drop to his forehead each day during his sickness. He was not cured, in the sense of physical healing, of course, but the hour of his death was little short of miraculous.

Neither Gill nor Anthony would see themselves as being 'religious' in any sense. But we know from their experience that it is love, not religion, which holds the key to the kingdom of heaven. This is one of the most important lessons we learn from Anthony's remarkable story; people do not get to heaven by being 'religious' but by learning to live in selfless love. When we turn to scripture we discern Gill and Anthony as participants in the story of God's people. The love of Gill for her suffering son is redolent of Hagar's love for her son Ishmael in the Book of Genesis. God, in compassion, acts to bring them relief from their tribulation in the desert:

For she said, 'Let me not look upon the
death of the child.' And as she sat over
against him, the child lifted up his voice and
wept. And God heard the voice of the lad;
and the angel of the Lord called to Hagar from
heaven, and said to her, 'What troubles you,
Hagar? Fear not; for God has heard the
voice of the lad where he is. Arise, lift up the
lad, and hold him fast with your hand.'

(Gen. 21:16–18.)

The Sleep of Peace

Anthony's final words to his mum, his last words on this earth, are brief: 'Mum, I can't hang on any longer. I can't do it any more.'

Gill, filled with sorrow as she realised that his last moment had come, asked her beloved son to close his eyes and to go to sleep; a sleep she knew would be forever. He bade goodbye to her, whom he loved most in this world; she, who had brought him into the world, had nurtured and cared for him the whole of his short life. Now, she watched him as he fell silent, closed his eyes, caught his last breath and took the final, momentous step on his journey. For a few moments, he had been able to grant her, by God's grace, a glimpse of the greatest mystery facing each human life. Now the veil was drawn, as Anthony's soul returned to the loving care of his Maker:

> In peace I will both lie down and sleep;
> For thou alone, O Lord, makest me dwell in safety.
>
> (Psalm 4:8.)

What are we to make of Anthony's last few brief words? What was implied by the apparently negative 'I can't hang on – I can't do it'? The essence of the message seems to be that he was in absolute haste to depart, that he must be going at once. There is an urgency in his words. Was he being pushed reluctantly away from this life by sheer exhaustion or was he being pulled away from it by the ineluctable longing to be in his new and glorious home? To approach an answer to this question, we must remind ourselves of our lines of reasoning about the nature of his revival at the hour of his death.

There is little doubt that his body seems to have been sustained, during the few minutes of the time he was speaking to his mother, by a power not of this earth. Immediately before his extraordinary and all-too-brief revival, he had been in a state of extremis and was clearly approaching the end of his life. His doctors, as we have seen, later confirmed that his condition precluded the ability to speak. His natural situation was grave, as he could scarcely breathe, he had no energy and his life-processes were failing fast. Therefore, his unexpected revival was, quite literally, beyond the natural. It was inexplicable in terms of the natural sciences. But all things are possible with God, as we have seen in His remarkable question to Abraham and Sarah by the oaks at Mamre:

> Is anything too hard for the Lord?
>
> (Gen. 18:14.)

If we suppose that Anthony's revival was brought about by the divine will, through the strength of the Holy Spirit, we may draw several inferences which may help us to understand his apparent sudden haste to depart:

- It seems that God willed that Anthony's brief revival should take place.

- Thus, there must have been a reason, or reasons, for this.

- When the strength sustaining him was withdrawn, we should expect Ant's physical body to collapse quickly, because of his pre-existing very weak condition.

- Divine intervention at the end of Anthony's life implies that his soul would certainly not be abandoned after his death.

The question we need to consider with respect to the second statement above is: why should it be God's will to allow such a confirmation of love and assurance from the dying son to his grieving mother? The answer must surely be that God wills such remarkable events out of the compassion and love, which are His very nature. Perhaps the greater the love between people, the greater is the suffering in grief and such poverty of spirit will attract His compassion and His will to act? If so, why does He not always act in similar circumstances? Perhaps He does and His ways are invisible to us. We cannot comprehend the mystery here, but as Jesus shows, we can be sure that God suffers with us. The source of our healing in tribulation appears to arise from the very wounds we (as part of humanity) have inflicted upon Christ. We are certain that God, who is love, does not will the terrible suffering we see in the world and we have the evidence of His Son's particular concern for the anguish of children:

> So it is not the will of my Father who is in heaven
> that one of these little ones should perish.
>
> (Matt. 18:14.)

Jesus is telling us that His Father will not let any child perish, that the souls of innocent children cannot be lost. Thus, we have the reason for what we caught a glimpse of. Anthony was not perishing, but he was being carried out of the suffering world into a new and everlasting life. Furthermore, in His mercy, our heavenly Father allowed this comfort to be communicated to those who had suffered alongside Anthony and who were now grieving over him. Why such a privilege was granted we do not know, but we who loved Anthony are bound to praise God for His compassion and we adore Him for the amazing bounty of His tender, loving kindness as He gently received Anthony's soul.

What has been said above seems to confirm an important insight we have mentioned before: namely, that God chooses not to be omnipotent in the present order of creation. Because of human sin and the broken nature of the world, God's will is not done on earth as it is in heaven. He rescues people from their suffering in this world by calling their souls to Him. He has given mankind the freedom to act in the world as they wish and they have generally chosen the path of selfishness and have ignored their Maker's love for them and thus, His will. In the Lord's Prayer, we ask for His kingdom to come and for His will to be done, on earth as it is in heaven. We do this, because we know that our troubles arise from the lack of love of human beings, who have free rein in God's creation:

> We know that the whole creation has been
> groaning in travail together until now; and
> not only the creation, but ourselves, who
> have the first fruits of the spirit, groan
> inwardly as we wait for adoption as sons, the
> redemption of our bodies. For in this hope
> we were saved.
>
> (Rom. 8:22–24.)

Having reiterated our consideration about Anthony's revival from torpor at this late hour in his life, we are in a better position to examine his final remarks to his mother. He says to her that he 'can't hang on any longer' and that he 'can't do it any more'. We have to consider what it is that he can't do any more and why he can't do it. The term 'hang on' suggests clinging to a place for some reason, but only with great difficulty and knowing that one will have to vacate it rather quickly. It has a geographical and a temporal connotation, as well as indicating the effort needed to remain in that particular place. The words 'do it' refer entirely to the strength of will needed and that in this case, continuing it is not an option. If our earlier inferences are correct, Ant could not keep going any longer in this world, because the strength he had temporarily been granted was now fading rapidly. He simply could not do what he was doing for his mum (to talk to her and to reassure her) any more, however much he might wish to. His fading strength was loosening his grip on the world and at the same time he was being called elsewhere; he had to depart in haste.

Consider the differences of nuance with respect to causation between the two statements: 'I can't hang on any longer. I can't do it any more.'

Both imply that Anthony has been making an effort to stay with his mother. Does not the latter suggest more urgency? We get here the sense that Ant feels it is he who is sustaining himself in this world somehow and now he no longer has the ability or strength to do so any more. The absolute certainty of 'I can't do it' brooks no interpretation other than that the effort or fortitude, mental or physical, required on his part is no longer tenable. What is it he can't do? Stay with his mum in this place or maintain the effort of keeping his physical body going? Probably both. This second statement tends to lean us towards the conclusion that he is reluctantly being pushed away from the world by his rapidly fading strength.

The first of Anthony's two statements, that he 'can't hang on any longer', suggests a slightly different interpretation. We feel that he has been holding on to his mortal life with difficulty for his mum, but that he knows he can stay no longer. He is, perhaps, almost apologetic, certainly reluctant. He also knows that his mum would dearly wish him to stay, just as he would love to be with her. But he cannot comply with her wishes, with her need for his physical presence. But why not; why must he disappoint her? The answer to this must be either that he no longer has the energy or ability or that he knows it is time for him to go.

I am sure that we have to accept both of these answers, but in doing so, we may be intrigued to wonder more about how he knew that he had to make further steps in his journey at this moment. Was he being called? At this point, we remember his companion, the lovely lady; she, whose very purpose was to guide him and to enfold him in love and security. Unfortunately, at this stage in his journey, we are not to know what thoughts or words passed between them.

Thus, although these two final statements have differences of emphasis, both are essentially telling us that he had to go. I have no doubt that his physical strength was at an end and that he was being called on his journey. We note that the timing of all these final moments in Anthony's life was under the control of powers beyond this world. For, although he was ultimately called with an imperative that could not be resisted, he had first been given the time and the strength to tell his dear mum exactly what it was that she needed to know. Now, in his haste to depart, surely he was pulled away from this world by the sheer attraction of the delights that beckoned beyond and by the impelling voice of love that was calling him? We have already discussed the excitement, the urgency and the fearlessness of Ant's initial remarks to his mum. Now, the amazing adventure that he was embarking on was there before him, he had to go, to be carried away into the midst of this divine experience that was expressly for him and for all the companions he loved.

This line of reasoning seems to fit the whole tenor of his remarks and it also lends credence to the idea (as suggested earlier) that the strength granted to Anthony came from the Holy Spirit. As he was called away on his journey, presumably the Spirit ceased supporting his body in the physical world and began to carry away his soul; his bodily strength would consequently fade rapidly. Though Anthony appeared to feel that it was his strength that was fading (his responsibility to 'keep going' for his mum), we always feel this of our physical and mental powers in the world. In fact, all the strength we have throughout our lives comes from God; for He is existence. We have every moment of our being through His mighty power. As Ant felt, in his desperate love for his mum, that he couldn't 'do it' any more, the truth is that it was not Ant's failure, or weakness, but God's will that was changing the very nature of this boy's existence. As he journeyed into his new life, with his lovely lady, he knew that he would always have his mother's love – he would not be separated from her.

A more prosaic explanation for Anthony's last moments would be to suppose that he simply found some remarkable final reserve of strength (perhaps because of chemical changes in the brain) and thus gasped out his farewell message to his mum. As his energy ran out, he was overwhelmed by terminal exhaustion; thus, his haste to finish his words. While this is possible, and indeed superficially convincing, so that many will believe it to be the only acceptable probability, the problem of his lungs throws considerable doubt on it as a persuasive interpretation. His physical condition was such as to forbid any words, let alone several sentences, delivered with urgency and excitement.

If Anthony was in haste to be gone, we are intrigued to know a little more about where he was going. Although our ability to make any progress in this fascinating line of enquiry is somewhat limited from our earthly perspective, we may gain a modicum of insight from the events and words leading up to his death:

- His entreaty to 'follow me', which he chose for his funeral, gives a glimmer of the excitement to come and of his ease of mind about the great adventure opening up before him.

- The vision of his beautiful 'angel' seemed to prepare the way for what he was to experience and to put his mind completely at rest.

- The urgency of his concern for his mother suggests the primacy of love in the world to come.

- The excitement in his words indicates that Anthony's spirit was starting to enjoy a fullness of life hitherto unavailable to him.

- His complete lack of fear as he is embraced in the love of God is heartening to us all. We should live in hope, not fear.

- Anthony's delight at being able to play with his 'superheroes' in complete freedom, and to be the centre of their attention, reflects the compassion of an all-knowing and all-loving Father.

- The glorious freedom that the separation of Anthony's spirit from his body appeared to give him helps to remove any doubts we may have about the survival of the soul after death.

- The faith Anthony placed in the 'lovely lady' who came to look after him shows that God's children are welcomed and cared for with tenderness and love as they leave this world.

All these aspects, and many more, serve to confirm for us the wonder and the love that awaits us at the end of life's journey.

One day, each one of us will actually follow Anthony on those final steps from this world into the next. As yet, we can only glimpse our pathway, 'as through a glass, darkly'. We can speculate about these incredible steps, as we have done with Anthony's story, and this is intriguing and encouraging, but to tread them ourselves, we have to be determined to make the right choice at every junction in the pathway. Anthony, in his brave journey, has done his best to point us in the right direction, but we must turn to the Word of God for the way, the truth and the life, for it is Jesus who holds the key to our salvation; He will teach us to grow in love, to pray, to fast and to give alms. He will ask us to be patient as we wait, with Him, in the garden, surrounded by the bewilderment, cruelty, violence and betrayal of the world, until His Father's will is done.

For the short time that he has been talking to his mum, it is as though Ant has been inhabiting two worlds; this physical world and another world beyond, a world we can only dimly discern. During this time, certainly throughout the period of his sickness and suffering, and before that, during the gentle innocence of his childhood, he has been making the gradual transition from this world to the next. What we have witnessed, perhaps, during his last moments, is the time of transcendence, when Anthony has hovered between life here and life elsewhere. We do not know when the process of going to the next world starts for Anthony or for anyone else. Our Lord might tell us that it starts at our baptism and gathers momentum as soon as we are devoted to following Him. Thus, the kingdom of heaven is able to start breaking into this world in the examples of individual lives. If we live in Jesus (in loving kindness), we can open a chink into the heavenly realm, as did Anthony for us, because we bring God, who is love, into the world.

Some people will start this heavenly transition early in their lives and they will maintain it as they grow nearer to God. Others may know it in the innocence of childhood and lose it again as they cease to grow spiritually, being suborned into the deceiving world by self-centred illusions of ambition, power and wealth that so often come with adulthood. (Thus, our Lord's entreaty to become as little children.) For yet others, the transition may be made suddenly, perhaps later in their lives or even on their deathbeds. Some, who cannot open their hearts, may never allow the healing love of God to reach them and rescue them from the destructive powers of this world.

For Anthony, a gentle and innocent boy, his whole life comprised this transition. His life was the journey, through suffering, that we are all asked by Jesus to make. To return to a question we posed in the chapter on The Gift of Anthony's Life, the promise of Ant's short life was fully realised and we have been given confirmation of this in his final moments. We believe the promise of Anthony's life was realised as he offered it up to God and it was accepted in boundless love by the One who had guided him on his journey, through pain and deprivation, hand in hand. The Book of Revelation gives a radiant image of the innocent in heaven:

> Then one of the elders addressed me, saying,
> 'Who are these, clothed in white robes,
> and whence have they come?'
> I said to him, 'Sir, you know.'
> And he said to me,
> 'These are they who have come
> out of the great tribulation;
> they have washed their robes and made them
> white in the blood of the Lamb.
> Therefore they are before the throne of God,
> and serve him day and night within his temple;
> and he who sits upon the throne shall shelter
> them with his presence.
> They shall hunger no more,
> neither thirst any more;

the sun shall not strike them,
nor any scorching heat.
For the Lamb in the midst of the throne
will be their shepherd,
and he will guide them to springs of living water;
and God will wipe away every tear from their eyes.'

(Rev. 7:13–17.)

Anthony's nurse Francis is quite clear that such deathbed pronouncements as Anthony made are not rare. He, too, sees them as evidence of the journey these children are making. Representing the spiritual journey, Francis uses the ancient symbol of the labyrinth, which is a complicated but regular pattern of passages, with many twists and turns. Unlike a maze, the labyrinth does not confuse and it has no dead ends. The journey through its winding paths allows time and solace for prayer and reflection. Only persistence and faith in the ultimate goal are required to arrive, eventually, at the certain destination. If our ears, eyes and hearts are open, we shall draw great comfort from the evidence of these spiritual pilgrimages made by children. Such revelations happen for a reason, which may not always be ours to know. But the closeness of children to God always, and particularly at their time of sickness and death, can scarcely be doubted.

The fact that Anthony said that he could not 'hang on any longer' (i.e. in that particular time and place) is confirmation that his soul was moving. These very words, far from being a cry of despair, inform his mum that he will be continuing his journey and for this to be possible, his lively and enquiring spirit will still exist. Though he had left his body behind, to be cared for by his loving mum and, in due course, to be committed to the ground in his little garden of remembrance, she knows beyond any doubt that his precious soul will always be with her.

Anthony's experiences have given us a glimpse of the soul's immortality. The beauty that can radiate from the faces of the exhausted and broken bodies of those at or near death, especially children, can be almost shocking in its power. At his death and after, Anthony's face shone with peace and happiness, a peace that was certainly beyond the power of this world. It was his final bequest of strength from his physical body to those many who came to grieve over him. In the beauty and calm of his face, his loving spirit shone through:

But I have calmed and quieted my soul,
like a child quieted at its mother's breast;
like a child that is quieted is my soul.

(Psalm 131:2.)

Anthony's body fell into the eternal quiet of his last sleep on earth in his mother's loving arms. He was a child calmed and quieted in the love of the woman who had given him everything. His soul slipped away in peace, in the certain knowledge that her love would be with him in the glorious adventures that now awaited him. Anthony's faith is confirmed by that of other brave souls who have faced their deaths with equanimity. It is certain that Ant would have admired Sir Thomas More who, at the point of his death on the block, said to his executioner, 'Friend, be not afraid of your office. You send me to God.'

Cranmer, who was standing nearby, replied, 'You're very sure of that, Sir Thomas.'

'He will not refuse one who is so blithe to go to him,' came the indefatigable response.

It seems that my dear godson, who also lost his life on this earth before his time, was equally blithe to rush headlong into the arms of his heavenly Father, who surely welcomed him with rapturous delight.

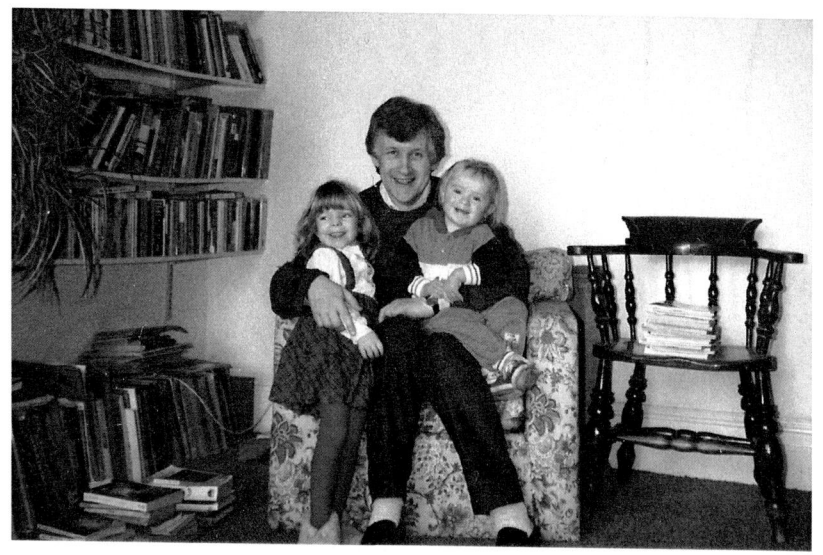

Katie (4 years) and Ant (18 months) with the author at Folkestone, 1988.

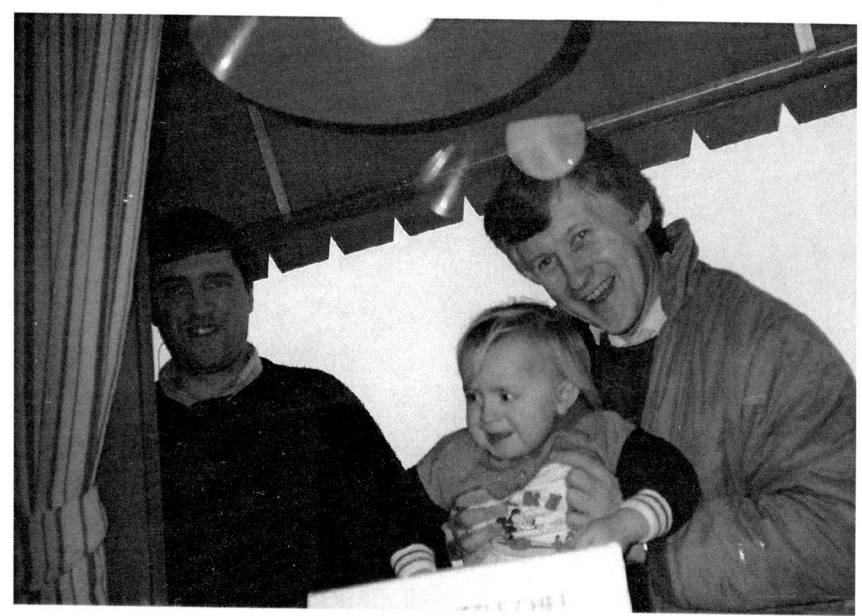

Anthony at 18 months with Michael (his father) and the author at Hythe, Kent, 1988.

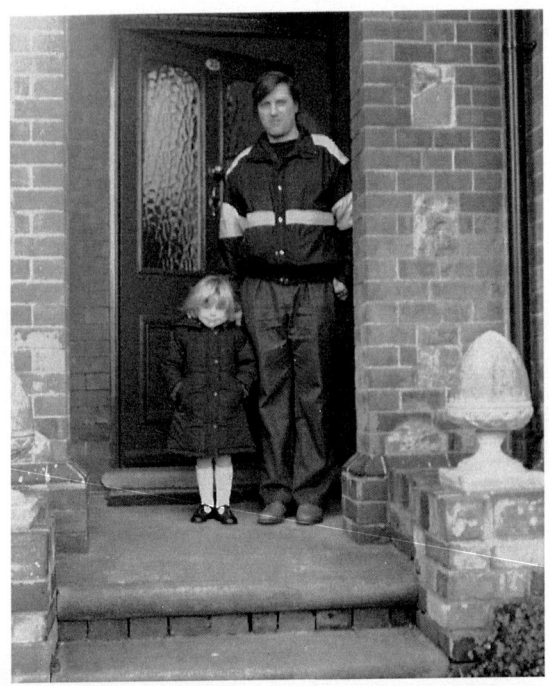

Katie (4) and Michael at Folkestone in 1988.

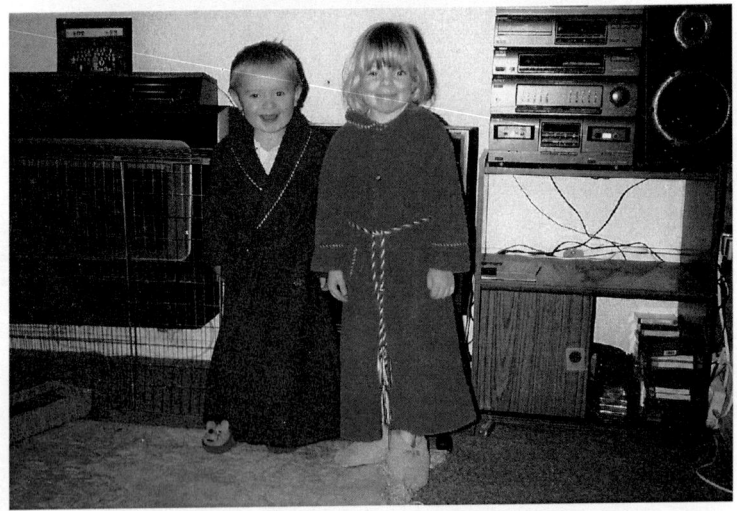

Ant (2) and Katie (5) ready for bed but wide awake, 1989.

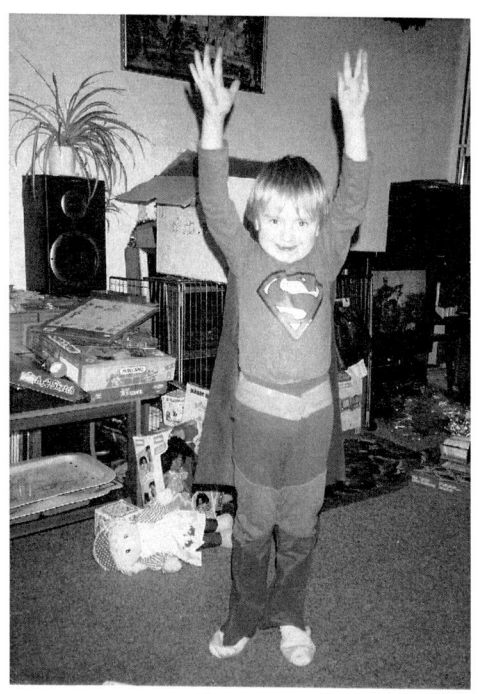

Super Ant (4) ready to take flight!

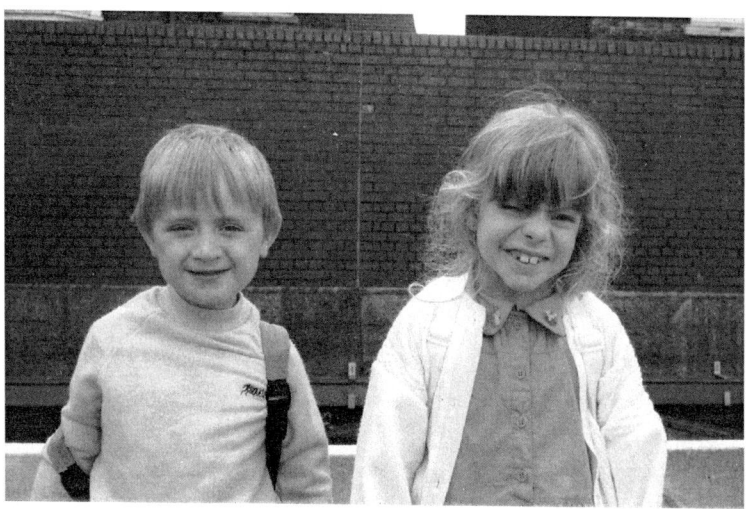

Anthony (4) and Katie (7) waiting for the train at Folkestone, 1991.

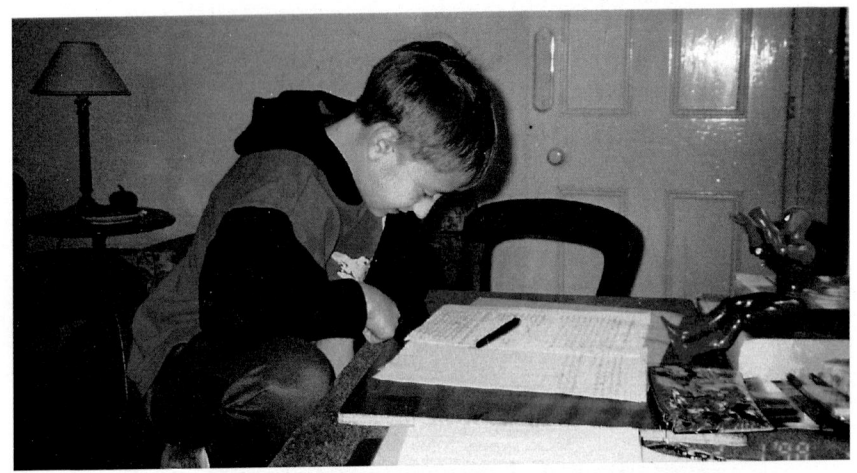

Ant (11) working for his Grammar School entrance exams under
Spiderman's guidance, 2nd January, 1998.

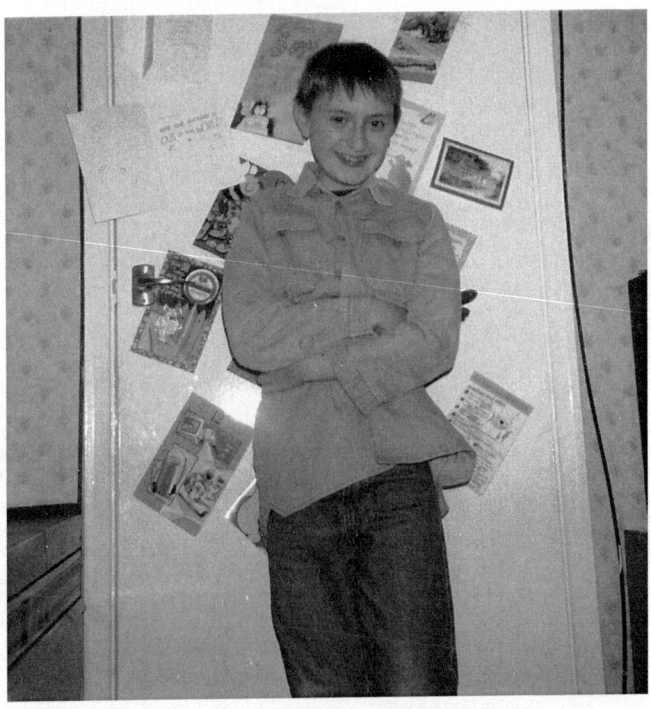

Anthony's 12th birthday, 28 December, 1998.

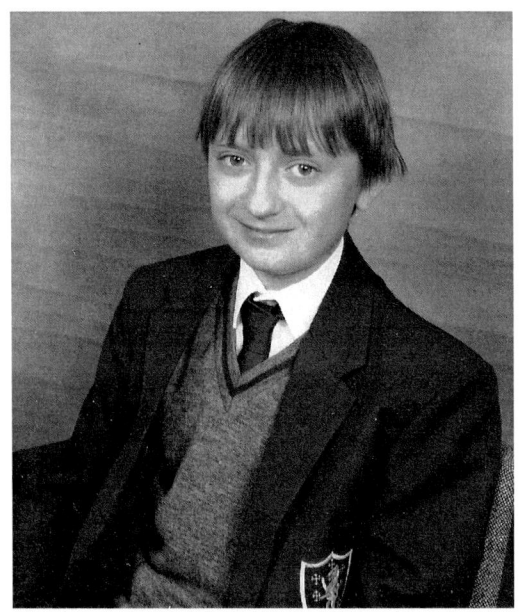

Anthony (12) in his first year at Lewes
Old Grammar School, 1999.

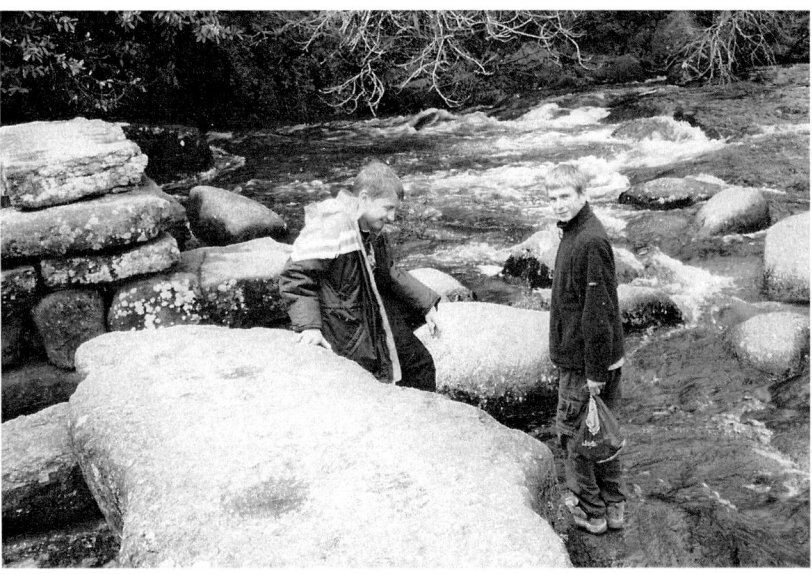

Ant and his friend Lewis (both 13) explore a stream in Devon, summer 2000.

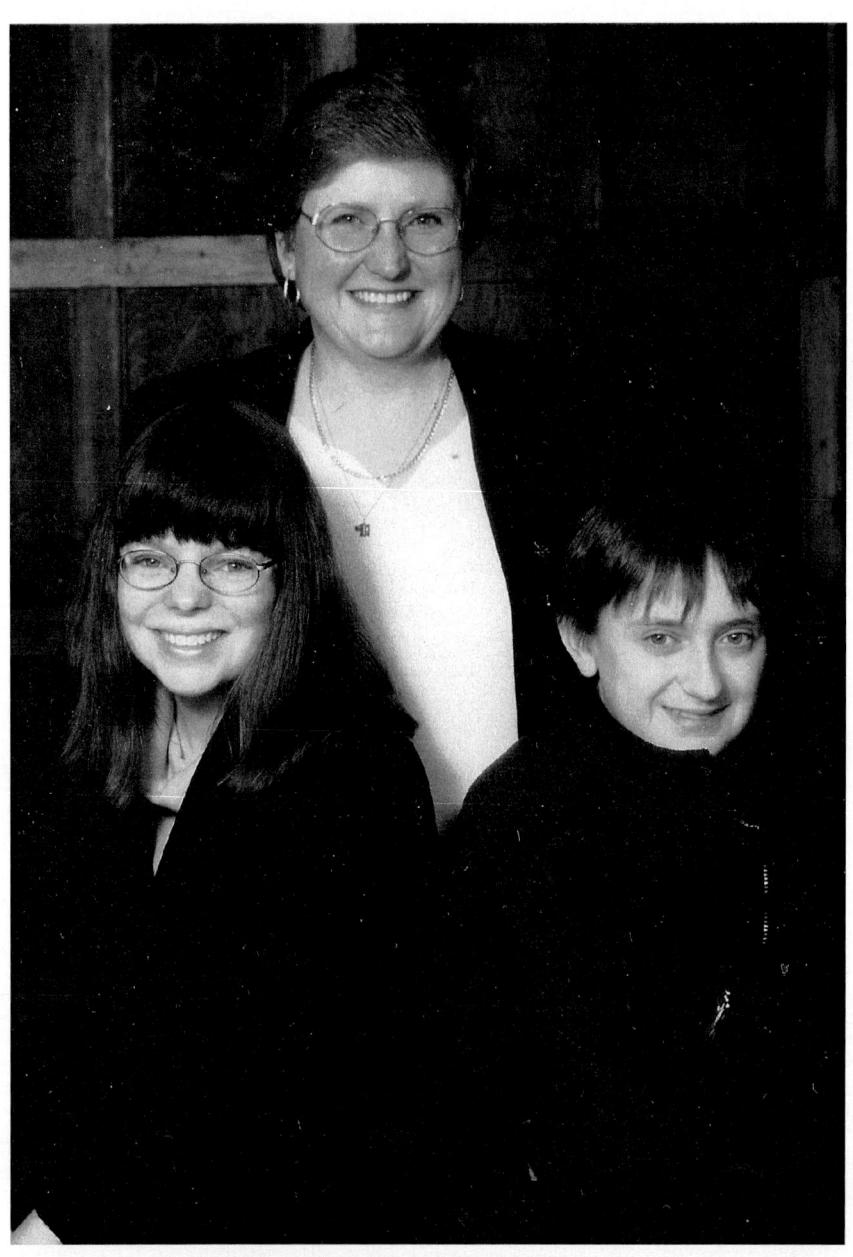

Katie, Gill and Anthony (14). Ant was unwell but his treatment
had not yet started. April, 2001.

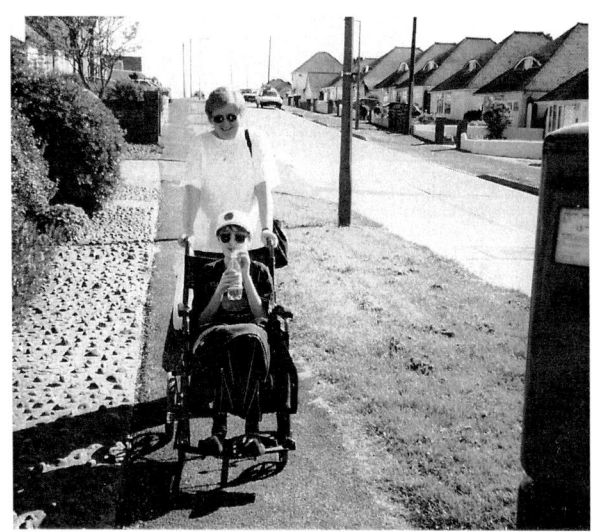

Gill takes Anthony for an excursion in Peacehaven during the recovery phase after his first chemotherapy session, 12th May, 2001. It was on such a walk thatAnt was greeted by the unknown boys (see page 15).

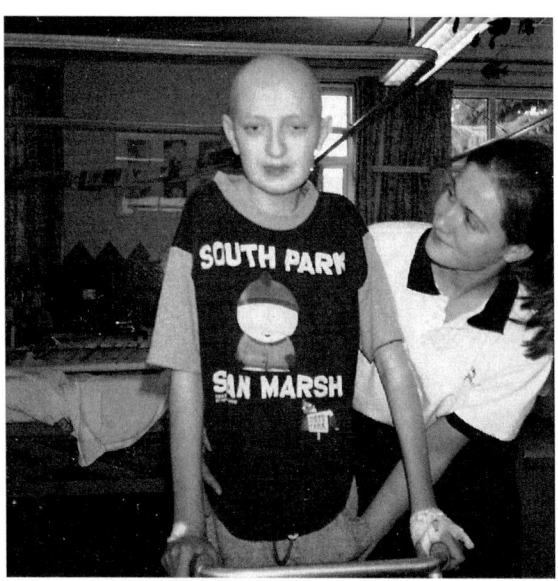

Anthony endures physiotherapy at Stanmore following the operation to remove his tumour, July, 2001.

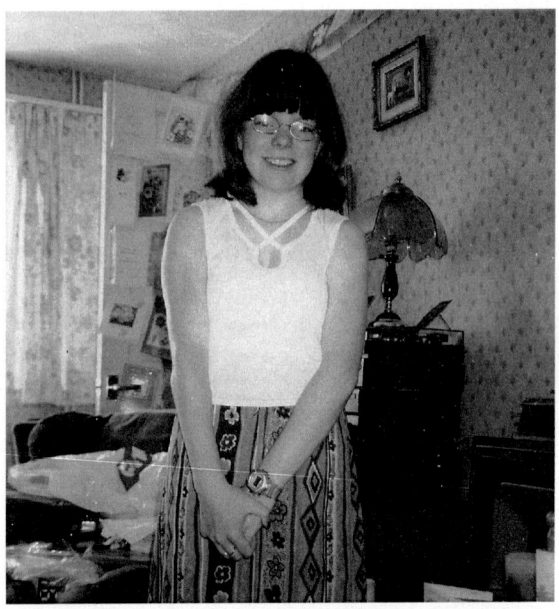

Katie (17). Anthony had just returned home following his operation and a long spell at Stanmore; thus the many "get well" cards, 16th July, 2001.

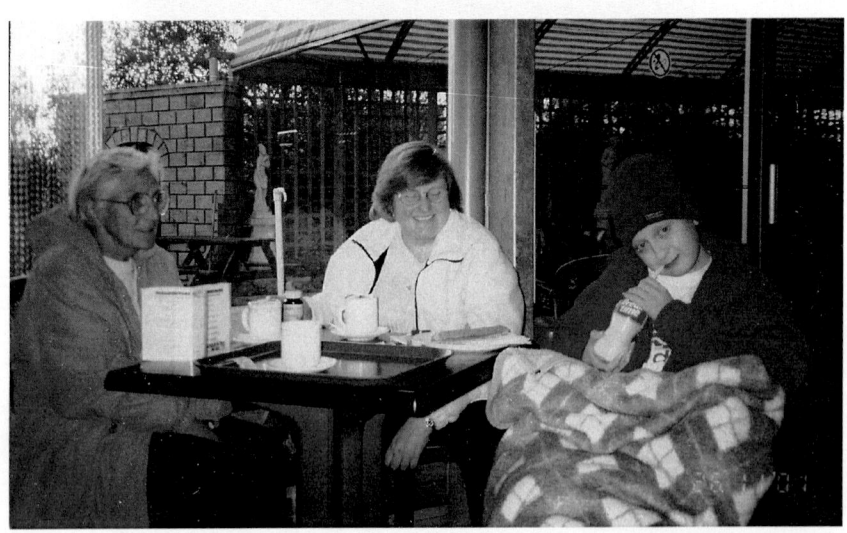

Nanny, Gill and Anthony enjoy a visit to Paradise Park, Newhaven, between chemotherapy sessions, 26th November, 2001.

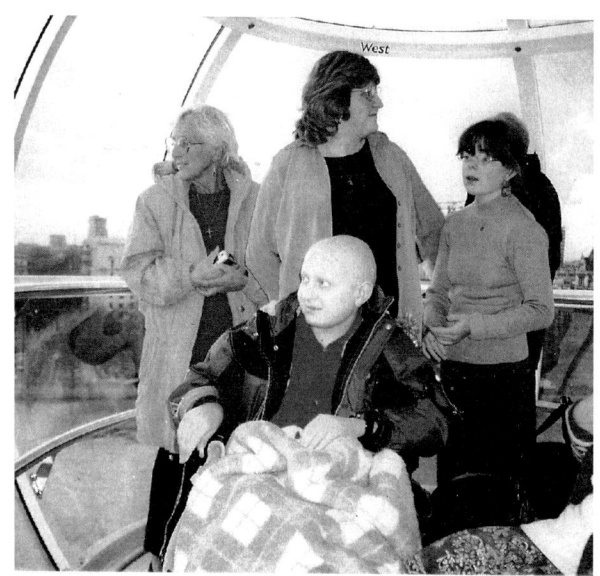

Ant and family are lifted skywards on the London Eye. In the rear are Nanny, Gill and Katie. 4th December, 2001.

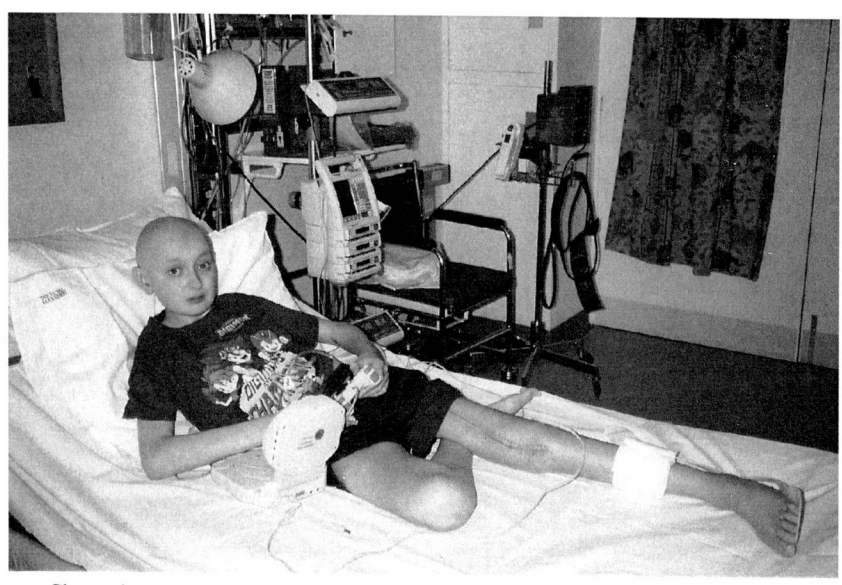

Chemotherapy at the Royal Marsden. Ant passes the time on his Playstation. By now he was a veteran of "chemo" – this was his sixth session. 15th December, 2001.

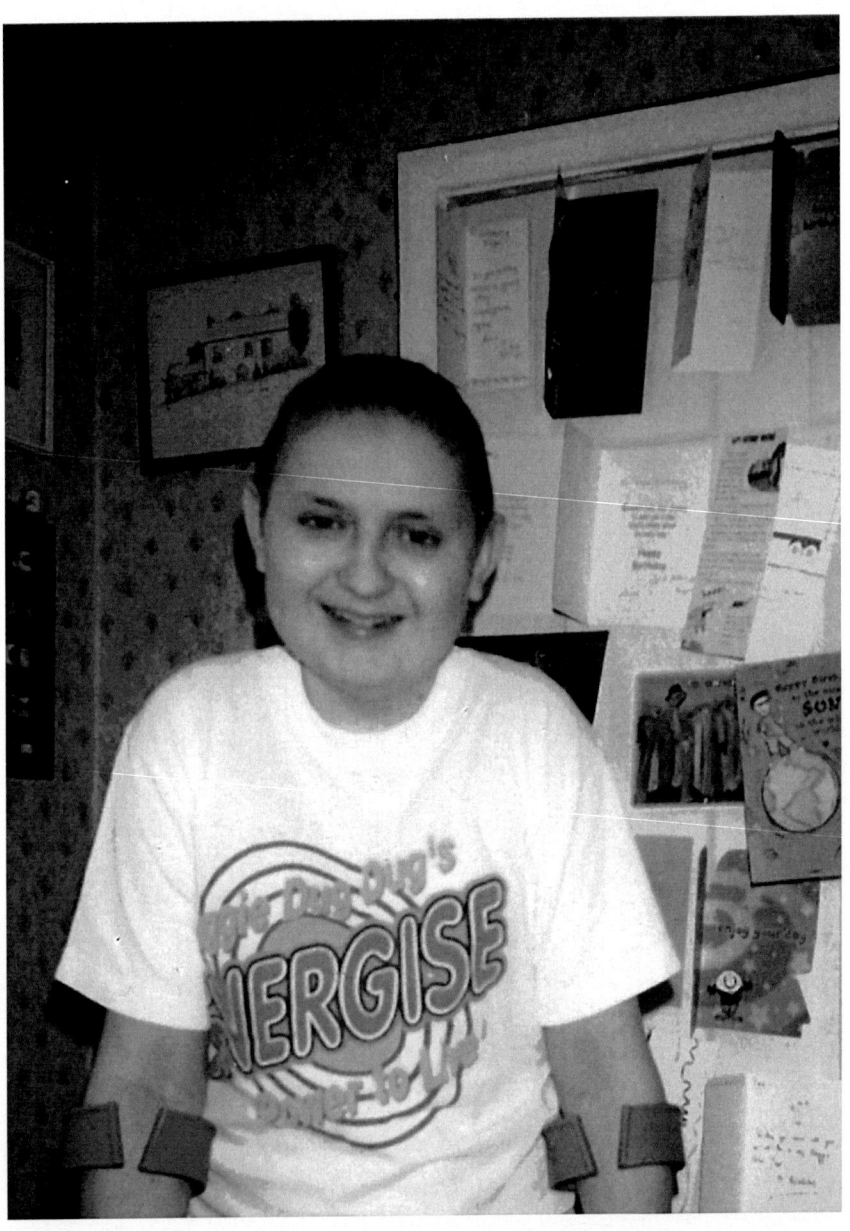

Anthony uses his crutches on his last birthday, 28th December, 2001. He was 15.
The effect of the steroids in fattening out Anthony's face is clear.

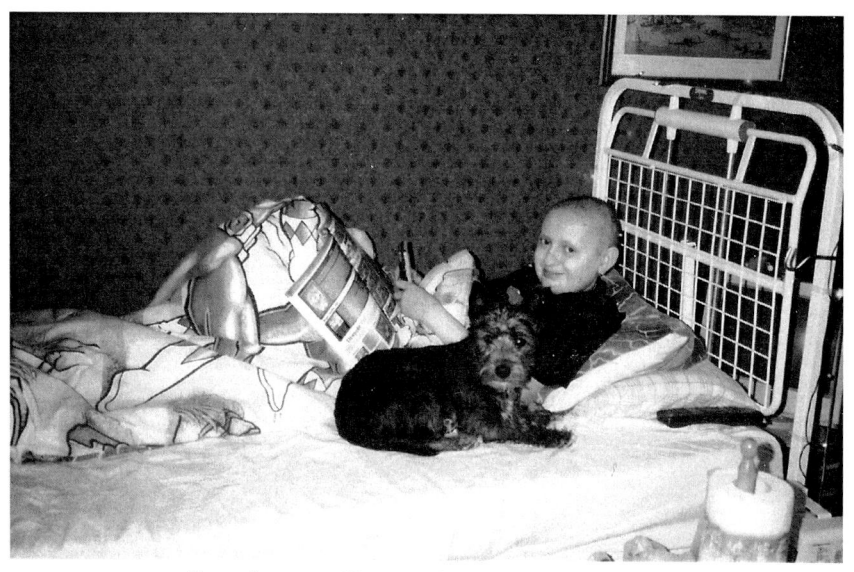

Toto takes care of her proud master, Christmas 2001.

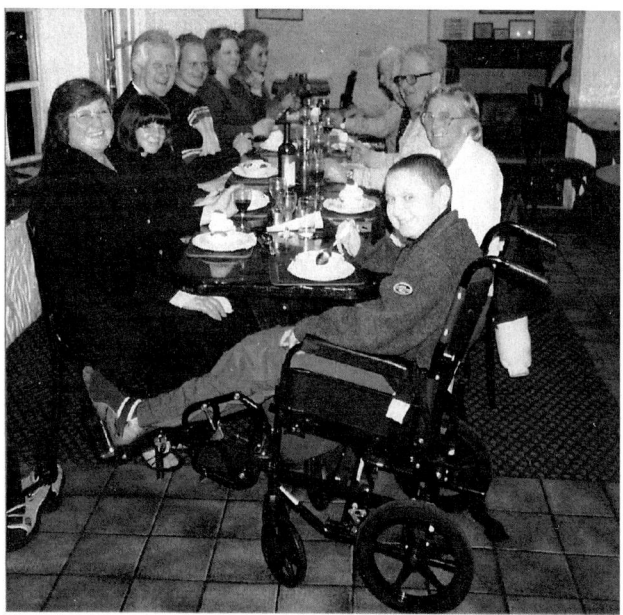

Katie's 18th birthday dinner. Left: Gill, Katie, author.
Right: Ant, Nanny, Grandad George. 8th March 2002.

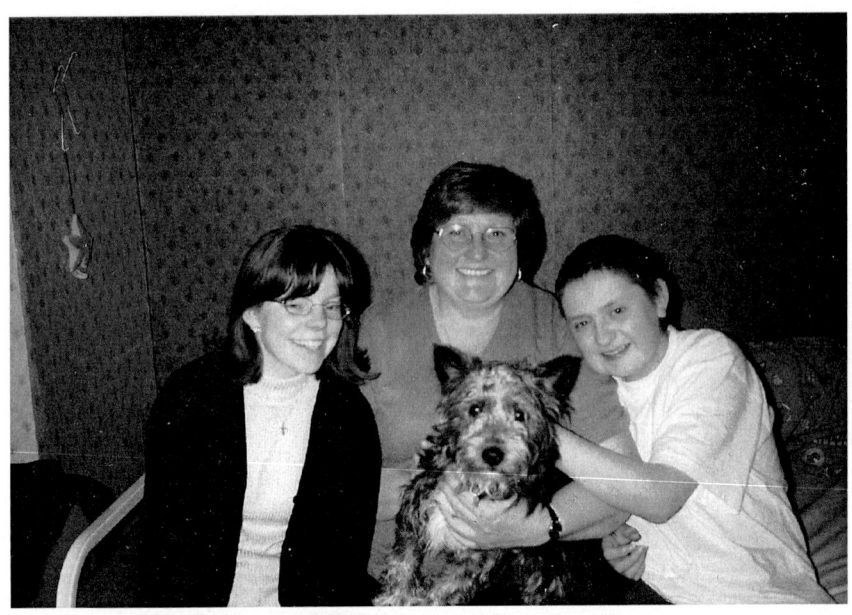

Toto hogs the camera, Gill, Katie and Anthony in supporting role, May, 2002.

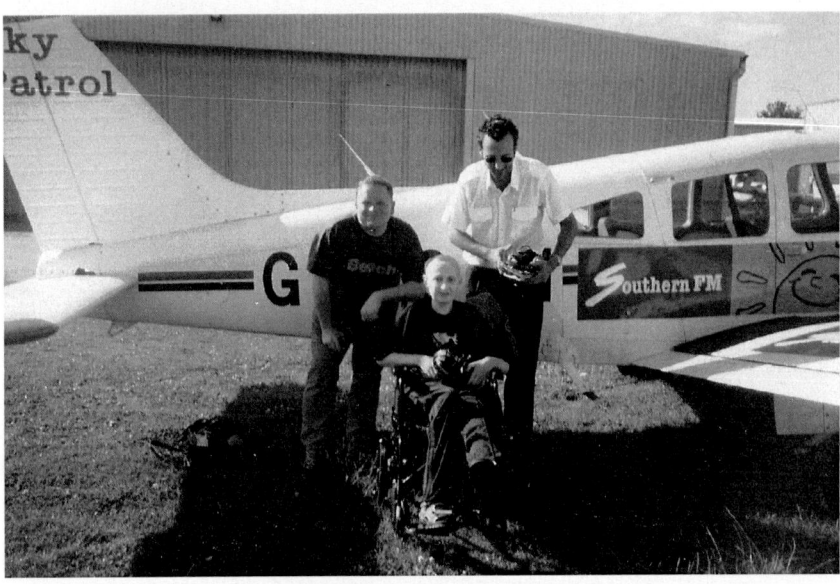

Ant prepares for his first ever flight, Shoreham Airport, 13th August, 2002.

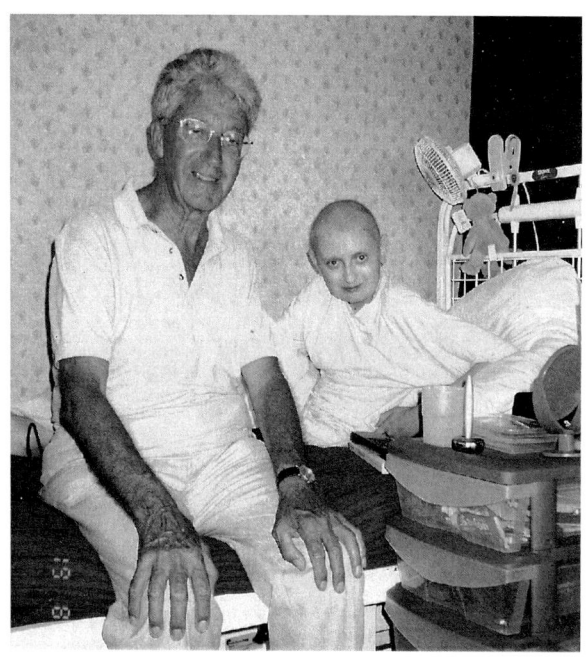

Anthony, by now very ill, with his paternal Grandad Tony,
19th August, 2002.

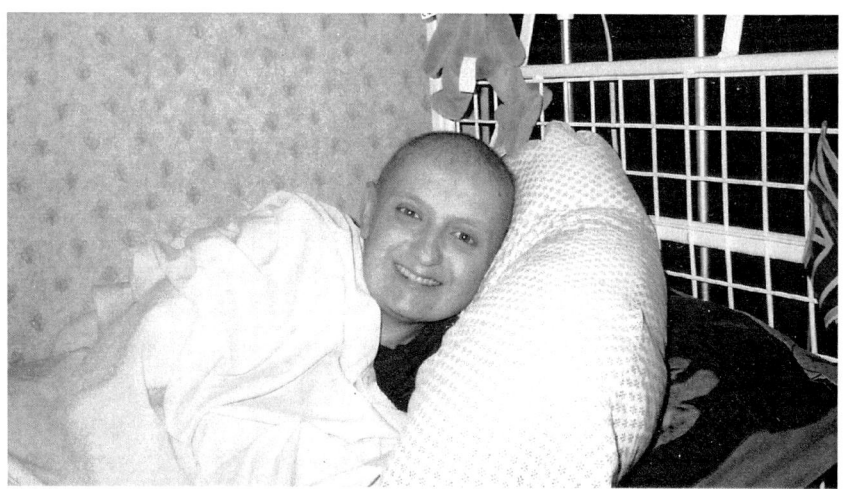

The author's last photograph of his godson. Now desperately ill,
Anthony still manages his beautiful smile, 29th August, 2002.

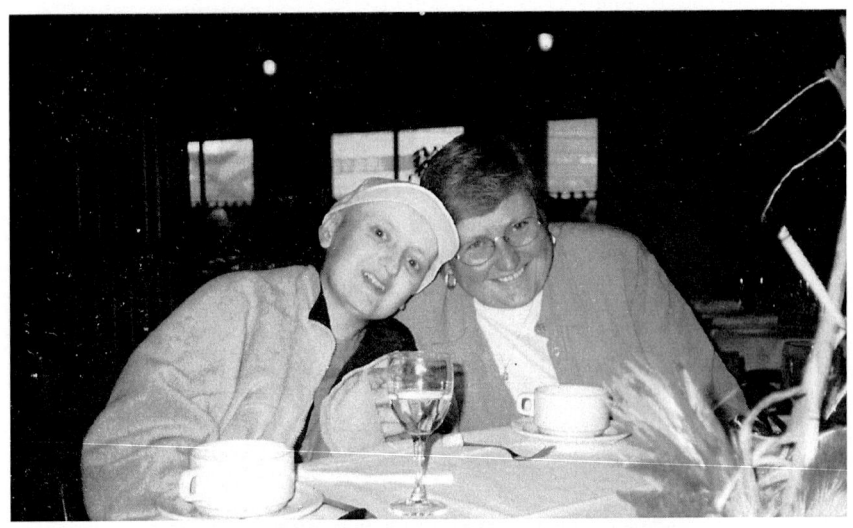

Ant and Gill confirm their unceasing love, September, 2002.
He had one more month to live.

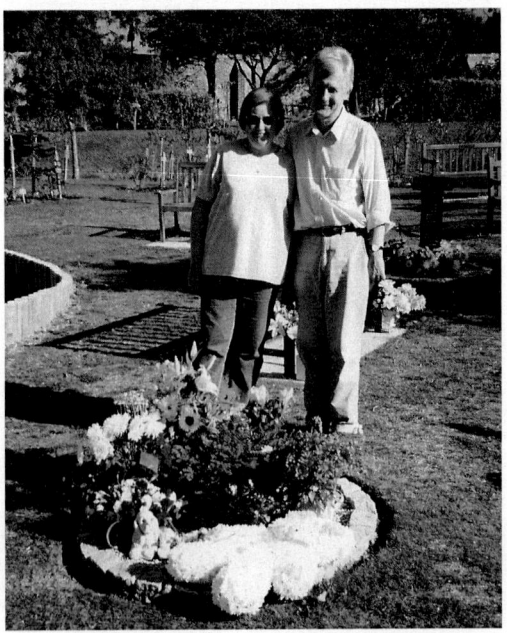

Gill and the author at Anthony's grave,
11th October, 2003.

Katie

Katie, Anthony's sister by adoption, makes a special contribution to our understanding of his journey. Her unique gifts grant us a privileged view of her brother's life and of his experiences. And through her dreams, Katie extends our perception of Anthony's journey even beyond the veil of death. Katie's entry into the world was difficult, as had been Anthony's. She was born on 8 March 1984 in Gravesend, Kent, to loving parents, who lacked all the other resources to look after her. Both of her parents were physically and mentally frail. Her mother had fallen on the stairs with an earlier child, so Katie was removed from her parents by Social Services and was put into the care of foster parents. There, she flourished in the love of a good family and was provided with an excellent start in life. She was adopted by Gill and Michael in 1985 and was over two and a half years old when Anthony was born on 28 December 1986.

Thus, within her first few years, Katie had known three homes. Shortly after her adoption, Anthony's birth meant that some attention was diverted away from Katie for, as we have seen, he was not well as a baby.

Both children attended the same junior school at Telscombe Cliffs, where they seem to have had different experiences. Anthony did well at school, because of his natural ability and curiosity. Katie had more difficulties and did not find learning easy. Eventually, she was designated as a slow learner. After this, her schooling was completed at St Anne's Special School in Lewes. Despite specialised teaching and smaller classes, Katie did not show much interest or aptitude in her academic studies. However, at St Anne's, she was much happier in the small groups and the dedicated teaching ensured that some attention could be given to her special needs. During her schooling, Katie began to show considerable ability at art, using a variety of media. In particular, many of her abstract paintings demonstrate a striking expression of form and colour. Before she left St Anne's, Katie obtained her GCSE in art, a source of great satisfaction both to her and to her parents.

Despite this, Katie's confidence in her creative abilities was not strong and neither was her motivation well developed. It was obvious in this and many aspects of her life that her self-confidence needed building, especially in the cause of improving her relationships with others. She felt most secure with older people, who generally accepted her and treated her with kindness. She got on well with her immediate friends at school, but with children, and later with teenagers, of her own generation, whom she did not know well, she was less sure. Because she tended to be hesitant with them, they frequently ignored her and Katie had few close friends of her own during her schooldays.

After leaving school, Katie decided to undertake a catering course at Lewes Tertiary College. Here, under careful tuition, she developed well and formed some good friendships. She enjoyed the course and became an excellent cook and kitchen manager. She understood about nutrition, about a balanced diet and about food hygiene and she put all she had learned into practice. As Katie's culinary abilities increased, many of her friends and family have frequently benefited from her cooking skills! At the end of her course, she gained her NVQ in catering. This well-deserved award and her whole experience at college have done much to boost her confidence. It became apparent that Katie had been a late developer in both her work and her social skills, for now she began to flourish. During her later years at college, Katie experienced part-time work in catering in a cafe and at various residential care homes. Although, to her disappointment, she was often given menial tasks in the kitchen, she gained much valuable experience and began to demonstrate her skills in coping with often difficult people.

Katie's personality is delightful; somewhat shy at first with strangers, she is naturally a most friendly and caring person. Once she knows you and is sure of a kindly response, she becomes quite a chatterbox. She has a wonderfully disarming smile and delights, more than anything, to be with people she knows and loves. She is absolutely loyal to her family, perhaps more accurately families, for she has re-established contact with the remaining members of her natural family, her parents having died many years ago. Katie is full of kindness to others and would not say an unkind word of anyone. She loves her mum with all her heart and she is particularly protective of her in the family's terrible loss.

This outline of Katie's development and character is important in Anthony's story because, as his sister, she lived with him all his life. Their father Michael having departed from the family home following his separation and divorce from Gill, Katie was the person who, after her mother, knew Anthony best from day to day. Katie loved him dearly, as he loved her. As young children, they were good companions, though their interests and abilities were very different. As teenagers, an ironic banter developed between them, as is often the case between brother and sister.

For such a young and vulnerable person, Katie has experienced much suffering in her time. The anguish she has known seems to be bound up with the development of her courage as a human being. Having lost her original family and her foster parents, she was adopted by Gill and Michael, where she has, to an extent, inevitably taken a back seat to her brother, simply because of the passage of events. At first, Anthony was not well as a baby and then both young children had to live through their parents' divorce. Katie endured, alongside her family, the many months of her brother's terrible illness, culminating in his death. This was an appalling blow for Katie as to the rest of her family and, like them, her life has been changed forever. Not long after this, her much loved grandad George also died. Meanwhile, through her contact with her natural family, Katie had been coming to terms with the reality of the loss of her natural parents and with the sufferings of other family members. Katie has borne all this with fortitude. She has wept and suffered alongside her mum, to whom she has been an unstinting support. She has lived through experiences not normally visited upon one so young or so vulnerable. I think, especially, of her resolution alongside Anthony in his desperate sickness, in hospital and at home; and after his death, of her bravery in bidding her brother farewell and finally coming through the agonies of the funeral itself.

Shortly before Anthony died, he told Katie that he wanted to have a little talk to her. She speaks of this with great reverence and it is obvious that she will always treasure Ant's particular words for her, offered so soon before his death. The very thought of this special little interview, one-to-one, between teenage brother and sister, during which Anthony imparted his love and his dying wishes and hopes to his only sister, is heartbreaking. To Katie, it brought the very real fortitude of her brother's love. The potency of Anthony's wishes for her own happiness and bravery and for her care of their parents, especially, of course, their mum, has firmly established in her values and priorities for the rest of her life. His assurances about his own future have set her heart at rest and they have convinced Katie in her steadfast faith. As with his mum, it is certain that Anthony's brave spirit will never leave Katie's side.

Katie's strength has been enhanced by what she has endured. Her intuitive understanding of people and her own integrity have made her a loving and powerful source of support to those around her. Most importantly, she seems able to see through the distressing circumstances of what has happened to the underlying reality. She has a vision of life which cuts through the inessential concerns of most of us. Katie can often see and know the truth because, in a sense, she lives on a different level in spiritual terms than many others. It is a higher level. This is a wonderful gift from God and, remembering the learning difficulties which Katie has faced, is a special blessing. It scarcely matters whether one had some problems in learning at school, when one is blessed with the loving vision of people's hearts that is Katie's gift.

Katie's faith is absolute. She loves Jesus with all her heart and in her innocence and concern for others, His love lives within her. In her vulnerability and open heart, she is clearly a child of God and with God. Although Katie was overwhelmed by the loss of her brother, she has lived through this grief, she has grown spiritually and she knows with absolute certainty that Anthony is alive and safe in the loving care of Jesus. Katie also knows that Ant is beyond any more suffering and that he lives in happiness. She understands that their mutual love will never die and that in the fullness of time she, Anthony and all their family and friends will be reunited in eternal love.

How does Katie sense all these things with such confidence? Without knowing it, she exemplifies the Gospel, which tells us that through the power of the Holy Spirit, God's kingdom is in the process of being established on earth. As we learn from the Beatitudes (Matt. 5:1–12), God chooses the weak and makes them strong in His holiness.

Since her brother's death, Katie does not forget Anthony and she does not choose to put him out of her mind. In some mysterious way, he dwells in her heart. He is a part of her; the gift of his spirit has been readily taken up by Katie. This has added to her confidence and her growing maturity. She is sure of their love; she understands its quality and its inviolable nature. Katie knows, with wisdom denied to wise men, that the only thing that matters is love. Where love is present, human beings become human – they become what they are meant to be. Where love is absent or denied, human beings destroy their very selves:

> For what does it profit a man,
> to gain the whole world and lose his life?
>
> (Mark 8:36.)

Katie is young and she will carry Anthony's memory with her during her own life's journey. We had hoped that, as the two children grew up, Anthony would live up to his responsibility of taking care of Katie, because of her academic weakness. Anthony's death seemed to leave Katie potentially exposed in a rather hostile, difficult and uncaring world. In fact, Anthony still takes care of her and she of him, but in a way that could not be foreseen. God's plans for us work in mysterious ways and the lesson for us is that we must learn to trust Him. Though we may feel powerless and lost, we should put ourselves in His care and let His will for us be done.

Katie talks with love of her memories of Anthony, particularly of the happy remembrances she has of the times they enjoyed together. She is not reluctant to talk of him and in many ways, he is still very real for her now. She has a large and treasured collection of photographs of her brother and these bring her much joy.

Remarkably, Katie's experience of her brother extends to her dreams. The perception of his incredible journey that Anthony was able to give us at the hour of his death is continued even beyond death by the glimpses Katie affords us from her dreams. Katie's dreams of her brother seem to occur from time to time, not at regular intervals, but certainly not infrequently. She says that she often wakes knowing that she has dreamt about Anthony, but cannot remember the details. Fortunately, she remembers some of them; two examples of which will demonstrate the vision that Katie has to offer.

Not long after his death, Katie said that she had met Anthony in a dream. She was surprised to find him well and happy, and walking. Her surprise is understandable, because she had been used to seeing him bedridden and desperately ill for the last eighteen months or so of his life. In particular, he had not had the full use of his left leg during the whole of his illness. Now, in her dream, she saw that he could walk and run again. She was, of course, overjoyed to see him in such good health and this has been the case in all her dreams of Anthony.

In this early dream, she told me that she was also surprised by what Ant had said to her. He asked her if she would like to see 'the dinosaurs'. She was rather taken aback by this question, as she had never particularly liked the idea of the dinosaurs, though she knew that they had been firm favourites of Ant's during his life. Katie told Anthony that she might be frightened, but he assured her that she would be fine. Delighted to be with her brother, she acceded to the idea, hiding her reluctance from him but heartened by the thought that he must be familiar with them, to be so sure that they would both be safe with such gigantic beasts.

Anthony led her through the forests and she followed with some trepidation until, eventually, they came upon the dinosaurs. Katie said that she was astonished, because they turned out to be very friendly. Anthony showed her how you could safely stroke them, feed them leaves and even play with them. Despite their size, they were very careful and would never hurt you. The adventure came to a remarkable culmination, when Ant took her for a ride on his favourite dinosaur. She said she was not at all afraid.

If we accept the dream for what it is, we can certainly rely on Katie's trustworthy account of what she experienced. She is always candid and sincere in her conversations with me and besides this, she would surely not wish to deceive in an account of an experience she obviously regarded as being so important, particularly since it concerned her brother. It seems to me that her integrity is confirmed by the sheer improbability of the story, especially when we take into account all we have been taught about the supposed nature of dinosaurs. Katie was clearly as surprised as we are, to discover in her dream that dinosaurs can be so amenable. I do not think for a moment that she was either capable of constructing such a story out of her own imagination or, indeed, would have wanted to tell any untruths about her beloved brother. It is possible, of course, that she may, at some time, have seen the film *Jurassic Park* with Anthony (he certainly loved it) and this may have inspired the dream. Nevertheless, I am sure that she actually had the experience of the dream. Another likely inspiration for such a dream is that this is one of the things Anthony would most have wanted to do. He had always been intrigued by the dinosaurs and an important part of their mystique, of course, was the fact that they were extinct. If he could have been given the actual chance to see them, to touch them and to be with them, he would have relished the opportunity.

Perhaps Katie's subconscious mind built this wonderful dream adventure to please her brother, because in the magical world of dreams she was able to do anything for him. This explanation seems quite probable; an attempt by Katie's mind to offer the best gift she could literally 'dream up' for him. On the other hand, perhaps there is an even more intriguing, tentative elucidation. Could we suppose that the possibility we have just outlined may have been reversed? What if the dream was a gift from Anthony to Katie? If such a thing were possible, he would surely wish to bring her into his new life, to show her how well he was and to demonstrate what a wonderful world he was now able to explore. We are not to know if such a thing is possible, but if it is, we might guess that Ant would try it. We can certainly believe that Anthony might well have been playing with dinosaurs in his new life. We know from his remarks to his mum, in his final moments, that he was given the wonderful experience of being with his 'superheroes'. There is the distinct possibility that Katie's dream intimates that God does not deny Ant the dinosaurs, either. In fact, it suggests the probability that Ant's every wish is granted by our Lord; the boy may be indulged in his every expectation. If this is the case, it seems that the heavenly celebration provided by God for His innocent children who have suffered is completely beyond our imagining. But we can believe this; the story of the prodigal son (Luke 15:1–32) confirms that God's love is boundless and unconditional and His mercy is infinite. As St Paul tells us:

> What no eye has seen, nor ear heard,
> nor the heart of man conceived,
> what God has prepared for those who love him.
>
> (I Cor. 2:9.)

The second dream to be related may add further credence to the supposition that dreams can enter our subconscious from elsewhere. On Monday, 3 May 2004, Katie spoke to me of her most remarkable dream to date. She began by saying that she had been dreaming about Anthony again. This time, he had shown her heaven. 'It was so wonderful, Ken,' she said, 'more beautiful than anywhere else I have ever seen.'

Katie described how, at the start of her dream, she was walking along a passage or pathway. As she moved nearer to the end of the path, she could see she was coming up to a little white fence. There was a gate in the fence and on the other side a man was waiting for her. As soon as she saw Him she knew He was Jesus. He had black hair and beard and He was wearing a long white robe. Katie passed through the gate and Jesus welcomed her with great kindness. He raised His hand and blessed her in the name of His Father, making the sign of the cross on her forehead. She could see the wounds in His hands.

Then Katie saw Anthony standing next to the Lord. Ant ran forwards to greet her and she saw, as in previous dreams, that both of his legs were healthy and strong. He was very happy to see her and he asked her about their mum. Katie said that he pressed her to continue to take great care of mum.

They passed into the loveliest garden you have ever seen. 'You would not believe how lovely, Ken,' said Katie. 'The colours of the flowers and trees were so beautiful, the sky was perfectly blue and there was bright sunshine all around. Little birds were singing.' Anthony showed her the small animals he had been playing with before she had arrived. Anthony then took Katie 'over all Jerusalem'. It was, she said, the loveliest place she had ever seen, with white buildings shining in the light and with peaceful gardens. The people were happy and kind and there was the sound of joyous laughter as children played in the sun-filled courts and gardens.

This dream has clearly made a deep impression on Katie. In a sense, it represents a vision of her faith, so it is a further foundation for the strength and integrity of her personality. We may see it as a gift of grace to this lovely girl. Katie concluded by confirming the depth of her faith, saying that she prays every day, thanking Jesus for her life and telling Him of her great love for Him and for all the people He has so kindly brought into her life.

I did not press Katie for any more details of the dream, as I wanted her account to stand exactly as she had related it. I simply accepted it and told her what a wonderful experience I thought she had been granted.

To say that I was amazed by this dream of Katie's would be an understatement. It is, in my view, another profound vision we have been given, as a result of the mystery of Anthony's death. As Katie related her words, I could scarcely grasp the depth and implication of what she had said. I knew these were wonderful words and because of this, they remained in my mind exactly as she had told them. It was only in the succeeding days, as I pondered over Katie's beautiful revelation, that the profundity of her experience began to take hold of my mind. What she said was so striking that it may be worth briefly examining some of the elements of her dream and considering their implications.

Katie was clearly struck by the beauty and wonder of what she had seen. She easily impressed on me the excitement and joy she had felt in the experience. The start of the dream consists of Katie's walk along the passage or pathway towards the little white fence. This introduction to her vision seems to be redolent of many 'near death experiences', in which people recall a journey through a passage or tunnel, representing the transition from this world to the next. The white fence also appears in some near death revelations. It is usually interpreted as indicating the boundary of the heavenly realm. Katie was certainly not aware of any link with near death experiences. She almost certainly does not know what these are. If she had known this, she would probably have been frightened, and she clearly was not. Her mood seems to have been one of excited anticipation.

Katie's expectation was rewarded as she beheld Jesus waiting for her. She recognised Jesus immediately. Significantly, He was standing on the other side of the fence, in heaven. Also significant was His black beard and hair. As Jesus was almost certainly, ethnically, a typical (and orthodox) Jew, His hair would most likely have been black, not fair as shown in most of our children's picture books. The authentic colour of His hair (unfamiliar to Katie from the usual pictures she would have seen), suggests the veracity of her dream and of her account of it. She was welcomed through 'the gate' by our Lord. She accepted His invitation and entered into the heavenly realm, where Jesus lives with the blessed saints. The symbolism of the gate is striking in what it suggests about the reward of grace Katie receives for her innocent love. She said 'yes' to Christ's invitation and was received. He invites us all and the answer we give depends on our love and faith. The kindness of the Lord and His blessing of Katie were obviously received by her with great love and they were just what she (and we) would have anticipated from Him. Although confirming and wonderful for her, she found His actions and words exactly consonant with what she would have expected from Him, because she had already recognised Him as the Lord. Katie noticed the wounds in His hands as He blessed her. Another authentic image (and utterly significant in the healing He was giving Katie's soul); His wounds were further confirmation for her, not that she needed any, that this was, indeed, the Son of God.

When Katie saw Anthony standing next to the Lord, she was struck again by the recognition that he had been restored to full health. He even ran to greet her. She accepted, without question, that Ant was the companion of Jesus. In fact, she would probably have expected to find him with no less a friend, following the suffering he had endured on earth. Anthony's concern for his mother rings true and was exactly what Katie would have expected of him. Her brother now led her on a journey full of wonder and beauty, the like of which she had never seen.

This final, descriptive part of the dream is, perhaps, its most remarkable element. Katie said that Anthony 'took me over all Jerusalem'. Her use of this name is quite incredible. She knew, somehow, that this heavenly place was Jerusalem. She had said at the beginning that Anthony had 'shown her heaven'. Katie, of course, has not read the Book of Revelation, describing John's vision of the New Jerusalem, which will form the home for all the faithful, where they will live with God in His new creation (Rev. 21:1–27). It is the most remarkable picture of heaven we have and we are struck by the close correlation between John's vision of the heavenly realm and this innocent girl's dream of it. Katie's awareness of 'the bright sunshine all around' is noteworthy, as is her expression of 'white buildings shining in the light'. Katie is struck by the intensity of the light; naturally, she accepts it as the light of the sun, but John tells us that it has a far more brilliant source: 'For the Glory of God is its light, and its lamp is the Lamb' (Rev. 21:23). Katie's vision of the overwhelming beauty and joy of the New Jerusalem, so similar to John's, is further confirmed by Isaiah's prophecy, where he, too, writes of God creating a new heaven and a new earth (Is. 65:17–25).

In her dream, Katie knew at once whom she had met and where she had been. It was the 'loveliest place she had ever seen', because there can be no lovelier place. How remarkable that Katie has already seen this place in her dream, having apparently crossed the threshold between this world and the next to do so. Of course, it is not surprising that Katie has been chosen to be the bearer of this wonderful message of love and hope. It is confirmation of what has been said of Katie, that in her kindness and innocence she is already with God. As our Lord tells us (Matt. 5:4–5): 'Blessed are those who mourn, for they shall be comforted. Blessed are the meek, for they shall inherit the earth.' It is my belief that Katie has seen the New Jerusalem, where Anthony now dwells in happiness, because her faith is complete. Thus, are all innocent children (young and old) beloved of God.

But there will be those, more sceptical, who will ask: but these were only dreams; how can we place credence on the content of mere dreams? The psychiatrist Scott Peck in his book *The Road Less Travelled* is certain of the importance of dreams in understanding the workings of the human mind. He reminds us that dreams arise from the unconscious mind, which comprises by far the greater part of the mind. The unconscious, it seems, guides and informs the conscious mind in many ways, not least in our dreams. It is as though the unconscious mind acts as a teacher and counsellor to the conscious mind. Jung called this 'the wisdom of the unconscious'. The unconscious seems to be a rich pool of understanding, a source of nourishment and succour for the conscious. This wisdom is also the origin of our consciences, which seek to check the wilder excesses of our conscious minds and therefore our wills.

Scott Peck speculates on how the grace of God may enter into our consciousness. He postulates that it may come out of the unconscious and one important manifestation of this may be in dreams; for the Holy Spirit may dwell in the unconscious mind. The unconscious, as the seat of all wisdom, may harbour the will of God. Thus, deep spiritual growth may result from profound meditation, in which the human soul sinks through the boundary between the conscious and the unconscious mind, deep into the refreshing wisdom of the unconscious. In this way, the soul of man may be healed and anointed by God.

Most dreams are beyond interpretation and, as Jung tells us, 'Dreams that form logically, morally, or aesthetically satisfying wholes are exceptional'. In these rare dreams that we can understand, perhaps we may experience the wisdom of the unconscious mind directly, because when we are unconscious, our minds are not disturbed so greatly by the physical world outside ourselves; few messages are being received from the senses. If we accept this psychiatric (and therefore scientific) understanding of the mind, we may begin to appreciate that dreams can yield information from the deep wisdom of the unconscious. If we also accept that the Holy Spirit may dwell therein, we may concede that dreams can be an important source of spiritual truth. It is possible that God dwells within our unconscious and that He may rise to communicate with us in dreams and in our consciences.

The Bible gives us many examples of God speaking to His people in this way. We think of Joseph's dreams and his interpretation of the dreams of Pharaoh (Gen. 42:8–9). Likewise, we remember Daniel's explanation of Nebuchadnezzar's dream (Dan. 2:1–11). Then there are the four dreams of Joseph, Mary's husband. All are messages to Joseph about the care of Mary and Jesus (Matt. 1:20, Matt. 2:13, Matt. 2:19–20, Matt 2:22). In each dream, Joseph is spoken to by an angel:

Behold, an angel of the Lord appeared to Joseph in a dream.

(Matt. 2:13.)

Dreams, as divine messages, have good antecedents and should not be lightly dismissed. Samuel Wells writes in his book *Power and Passion*: 'Dreams in the Bible are an inbreaking of God's future into the unpromising circumstances of the present ... they simply draw back the veil between earth and heaven, disclosing the purpose of God, and the mysterious ways God's purpose takes shape in the lives of his people.' We certainly should not ignore Katie's dreams. She is opening our hearts to spiritual truths, no less than did Anthony in his final words. Furthermore, in her intuitive understanding, she shares with us a view of the next world that might otherwise be unavailable to us.

Katie gives us a remarkable gift. She adds to the wonders Anthony has previously shown us and she confirms in her dream what we already knew but hardly dared to accept. The place where he dwells is the house of the Lord.

It is Katie's closeness to Anthony that allows his continuing presence to her. She teaches us a fundamental lesson about the nature of love. It is not ideologies, principles, organisations, mission statements that we are to love, but people. We cannot have relationships with ideas, only with people. We should not live completely in an abstract world of ideas, but in the real world of people, because ideas can never be more important than people. (By people, we are talking of individual lives.) If our political leaders were able to see this truth, wars would be no more. We must be present to those we love; we support them; we give ourselves to them. It is in the tangle of our loving relationships that we find our humanity, our purpose, the value and the meaning of our lives. And it is Christ who, in filling our hearts and souls with His loving presence, grants us the strength to be human, to be at one with Him and to be all for those we love.

It is appropriate, since I am writing of my dear god-daughter, to conclude this chapter on an amusing and hopeful note. One day, when Katie and I were looking at the birds in the garden, Katie asked me which my favourite bird in the world was.

'The dodo,' I said.

'Trust you to say that,' replied Katie. 'Well, Ken, when you go to heaven you will have to ask Anthony to show you the dodos.'

As usual with Katie, when talking of spiritual things, this was said with absolute confidence, candour and conviction. I look forward to seeing the dodos with Anthony one day, before too long.

> I thank thee,Father, Lord of heaven and earth,
> that thou hast hidden these things from the wise
> and understanding and revealed them to babes.
>
> (Matt. 11:25.)

Anthony's Gift of Life

Anthony's life in this world was a gift to those who loved him. But as he crossed the threshold of heaven he brought the mystery of his person, all his qualities, all his response to the world, before his Maker. For when we die on this earth we make a gift of our lives to God. He gives each of us His gift of life and it is His word that sustains us in life from second to second. We make of our lives what we can; God gives us the choice for better or for ill. It is as though we start with a blank sheet, a *tabula rasa,* and we write on it as we may. When we die we return God's wonderful gift to Him. No doubt He will look with loving concern at the way we have invested the talents He has given us.

Jesus expounds this in His parable of the talents (Matt. 25:14–29). In summary, three servants are given talents of different value by their master. He then departs on a long journey and the servants invest their talents with different degrees of wisdom. When their master returns and the day of reckoning comes, only the two servants who have made a good profit on their talents 'enter into the joy of their master'. The third servant, who failed to make a return on his master's investment, loses all. The lesson of the tale is that we must use wisely the gifts God has given us. It is worth taking risks with the investment of our lives for the reward of our generous Master, in the light of the certain knowledge that He will return to reclaim His investment in us. The investment He talks of is, of course, His love. We know that with our lives, and with the help of His grace, we can make a contribution to the coming of God's kingdom into the world. He will support and sustain His children as they use the gifts He has given them for His sake. The loving choices we make and the risks we take with our lives for Him will be rewarded in full when He returns to us.

We also make a gift of our lives to those we leave behind. What worthwhile legacy shall we bequeath to those who have invested their love in us? What love do we leave them? What lives have we touched and changed? Have we chosen personal security by not risking our talents for our neighbour or have we thrown caution to the wind and given of our love, effort and skill to others, to try to make the world more of a reflection of His kingdom? Loving to the full, as God asks us to, means taking risks. But this is often the only way to invest the talents He has given us, to enrich the lives of those we leave in the world.

In considering Anthony's gift of his life to his Maker and to us, we can only do so in relation to the eventual gift of our own lives. What can we possibly return to God who has given us the gift of life itself? What, if anything, of eternal value shall we leave behind for those we have met, accompanied and loved on life's journey? These are questions for each individual to ponder over.

When Anthony died, his most important act was offering the gift of his young life to God. In the short time allowed him, he had completed his journey, having made a fine return on God's investment in him. By our Lord's grace, Anthony was able to show us that, at the hour of his death, he entered into the joy of his Master. We have absolute confidence, supported by all the evidence we have seen, that his brief life on this earth was an abundantly acceptable gift to the Creator of the universe:

- He lived in God's love; he was loving, friendly and kind.

- He put others first and he showed concern for those who suffered.

- He was beloved of his family, friends and school.

- His sense of fun was contagious and was with him to the end.

- He loved God's creation in all its aspects.

- He was creative and busy, never lacking for interest or occupation.

- He suffered with great bravery during his terrible illness.

- He was innocent and undeserving of any tribulation.

- His love and concern for his mum lasted to his final breath.

- His life was short, but he still brought home to God a rich harvest.

In what sense was Anthony's life a gift to us? His great legacy for those who knew and loved him is that the nature of his life and the manner of his death hold out promise, hope and guidance to us. He says 'follow me' and he points the way for us. We learn to look at the world through the eyes of innocence. We are brought face-to-face with the essence of suffering and grief. We look at our faith in God and our desperate need of redemption, love and hope. We face our own mortality and we are hastened to act by the remembrance that time is short. We draw from Anthony's journey, the strength and resolution to seek to bring home to God the gift of our own lives, as a return on the talents He has bestowed on us. In this chapter we shall consider some of the specific strengths Anthony leaves us as the gift of his life.

We return, first, to the qualities of mind that Ant showed at the time of his death, namely to his urgency, his excitement and his lack of fear. These are valuable gifts to us as we seek the way to make our own lives acceptable to God and to our fellow human beings.

We need to have a sanguine urgency in our lives, because every moment is a precious gift to us. Of course, there is no point in living in a state of neurosis as we desperately try to get through the complex agenda we have set ourselves, to extract the maximum value from each day. This is not the kind of urgency that will transform our lives. What we beheld in Anthony was rather an urgency of priority. We must choose to give each moment to doing what is best. It is our judgement of what is best that is crucial. Our dogged sense of urgency is, in fact, the gentle nudging of the Holy Spirit to make the right choices, so that we may help to make God's suffering creation a better place. This is what we were made for – to do God's will, to bring it into the world, where it is so desperately needed.

We must never forget what we can do for those who are suffering, for those we love, for friends and acquaintances and for all those we meet by chance in our daily lives. We knew, with Anthony, that God was within each precious smile, each helping hand and every kind word; from Ant and from those who cared for him. In the urgency of our priorities we see that the human spirit is made in the image of God's love. In our own lives, our sense of urgency, the urgency that is the gift of God's grace, must be to play our small part in putting the world to rights. That is what Anthony wanted to do as he took risks in his help of his friends. And that, in the end, is why God has given us life.

As we set about the tasks we have been given in our own brief lives, if we see the truth, as Anthony saw it, it is inevitable that we shall be filled with excitement as we enter into the beauty and wonder of the world created for us. It was a fundamental principle of Ant's life that creation was made for our delight and for our inspiration, not for our exploitation. As we have seen, he used the imagination that was God's gift to him to build his own delightful and magical realms, inspired by the wonders of the natural and man-made worlds and designed to right the wrongs he saw in life. As he was a child, he did thus in his fantasy; who knows what he might have achieved as an adult? By the grace of God, we each have the potential to transform the world, however infinitesimally, falteringly or intermittently, and in doing so, though we may not realise it, we transcend the boundary between the mortal and the eternal. As we try to do what God asks of us, He moves nearer to us. We may not think we can, but if our hearts are open, we will notice the mystery and wonder of His approach. Anthony's experience shows us that nearness to God brings excitement, love and peace.

And, of course, like Anthony, we no longer have any fear for our own future (however bleak it may appear) or for those we love and treasure. We know that, in the end, we are safe in the promise Christ has given us. We are filled with compassion for those of our fellow travellers who have suffered so tragically during their journeys through life. But the vision that comes with our faith gives us the strength to support and guide them. We remember that Ant, in his physical weakness, had no fear and he still managed to find the strength to inspire and to guide us. Fear vanishes, because we know that we do not depend on our own strength, or on the gifts the world offers us, but in an unconquerable strength and a priceless gift of faith. We are fearless, because we travel sure in hope and love; we accept the labyrinthine path of life's journey, because we are certain of our destination.

Anthony's life, which was to be so short, demonstrated his remarkable love of living. He used every moment to the full; it was almost an expression of an inner understanding that he knew each moment to be vital. He understood how he wanted to spend his time and he appreciated that there was not a minute to be wasted. He lived for the moment and in the moment, seizing the day and squeezing every ounce of discovery and creativity that could be had from it. In this way, he accepted God's wonderful gift of time, so freely given and so often squandered by many. It was almost as though he sensed that his time would be short and that he could not afford to lose any of it. Furthermore, he enjoyed to the full the gift of life he was given and he was even determined to do his best to continue enjoying it during his time of tribulation. He was particularly careful not to waste time, either in laziness or unkindness. If at all possible, he would avoid merely routine and mundane activities and would hasten through his school homework to maximise the time available for the proper employment of his own talents! For Ant, God's wonderful gift of life was there to be treasured and turned to fullest account.

How did Anthony use the time he was granted to employ his own talents? He did not simply use the opportunity; he invested it as God would wish him to. He took the gifts given to him and used these to make real his imagination; to enhance his world, to build, even in his little way, on the example of God's bountiful creation. He loved, and was intrigued by, the surrounding creation and its mysteries. He was keen to explore and to seek understanding of all the wonders available to him on this earth and in the heavens above. In this, of course, he was at one with many young people and he enjoyed joining in the voyage of discovery with his friends. Many were the sparkling conversations they had in those bright and promising days of youth; the dawn of exploration, the first footsteps into the beckoning mystery of the labyrinth of life's journey.

Anthony put his creative mind to work by using the gift of his imagination, together with the building blocks provided by the world of nature and the world of human beings. He was well aware of the timeless struggle between good and evil that has been an inseparable part of the history of humanity. Using his own imaginative skills, he gave life to his particular mythical worlds, filling them with detail, excitement and fun and bringing to the task every ounce of his mental and creative abilities. In a tiny way, Anthony reflected the creativity of his heavenly Father, as should we all. How else are we to invest the talents that have been given 'to each according to his ability' (Matt. 25:15), if not creatively, with imagination and with risk?

Anthony shows us that we must learn to see the world through the eyes of a child. To do this, we need to strip away the routine, the bureaucratic, the banal and the over-serious, leaving the fun, the grace, the love and the warmth. Such an approach is holy, because it is what God asks us to do, and with it love shines through the most difficult situations. Children can conquer the terrors of illness and death, because they know what is important; what they can see are eternal values. As children suffer, they are at one with God. He comes to them in their weakness; He treasures them, He stays with them. He fills them with His holiness, which may flash from their heavenly faces. As we weep over them in our compassion, our love and our helplessness, we easily forget that God is love and He is compassion. If we wonder where He is when we need Him in the depths of our despair, and why we cannot see Him, we need only feel the warm sorrow of our own tears. For as much as we have these virtues of love and compassion, we have them from God; He is within us in our tribulation.

As Anthony suffered and died before us, those who loved him were brought face-to-face with grief, as in helplessness, we beheld the suffering of our beloved and innocent child. This, too, in a bitter-sweet irony, was his gift to us; he brought us face-to-face with the very meaning of his life, with its value and its purpose. We believe that our Lord held Anthony in His arms and lifted him up to us, during his suffering. We were to look at him and to know the truth. In the mystery of grief, with our tears came the tenderness and humanity of Christ, bringing warmth, love and strength. From Anthony's death, we who loved him and love him still, as we yearn for his presence, can testify that grief is a healing gift, the balm of the Son who suffers with us.

Our society seems to encourage the delusion that it is possible to get through life in entirely favourable circumstances provided, of course, that one has the financial means to acquire all the necessary material possessions, facilities and services. The market place presses upon us the 'solutions' to all our problems. We know that all this is nonsense, no more so than when we lose a person we love. If we are honest with ourselves, we also know that suffering is an inevitable part of life. We cannot elude grief and if we attempt to do so, by holding it at arm's length or by hardening our souls to resist it, we shall merely devalue our own humanity. We have only one option and that is to kneel before our Lord and surrender to the grief He offers us, for grief is a gift from God. This is a paradox that is very hard to accept when we are suffering in bereavement. But the one we grieve, and whose presence we crave, also longs to be with us. When we surrender to the transforming power of grief, we can be brought, in the depth of our love, nearer than we have ever been to those we believe we have lost.

We must set aside the 'solutions' our world seeks to offer: 'closure' (the packing away of grief, boxing it up, so that we can escape from it) and 'coming to terms' with our loss (as we attempt to take control of the situation, thereby denying God's healing salve). Trying to forget grief, by busying ourselves with work or by changing our lives in some way, in order to 'get over it', is simply avoiding the healing balm that God provides for us. He alone knows the needs of our souls and He is the only one to whom we can turn in our distress. The richness of grief, the truth that is so often hidden from us as our hearts break for the loss of those we love, is the very way we offer the gift of ourselves to those who have died. The agony of our souls is a measure of the gift of love we bequeath to those we lose in the world. We see that Anthony's gift to us is balanced by our love for him in the incomparable, mutual adoration of bereavement.

As we grieve, we move close to God in the depths of the mystical relationship between suffering and love. Our nearness to Him in our grief allows Him to heal us as, with His gentle touch, He binds our broken hearts. We must learn to live through our grief, allowing God to change us as He wishes. For we, who loved Anthony, know that the experience of grief will change us forever. We shall be different people, because we shall have a new perception of reality. Friends of mine have already told me that I am not the same person that I was. As it is God who has touched us and changed us, whatever the alteration in us, we know it is what He wills. His will has been done on earth as it is in heaven.

The sadness of grief will yield eventually to hope. The mortal body decays at death and returns to the earth. But the spirit, carrying the soul, the centre of our being, passes from the temporal world into eternity. Our hope rests in the incredible promise of immortality made by our Saviour. It is the promise at the heart of our faith:

Truly, truly, I say to you,
if any one keeps my word,
he will never see death.

(John 8:51.)

We have been shown, by grace, through Anthony's remarkable experiences at his death, and by Katie's amazing dreams of Anthony's adventures in his new world, that life after the death of the body is surely part of God's continuing miracle of creation. Anthony was fascinated by the wonder of existence; by the mystery of life and by what may lie beyond the universe of our limited perception. He wanted to know so much and now, I am sure, he delights in wonders beyond our comprehension.

Anthony is but one of countless numbers of children who have suffered and still suffer in the world. His story has been our specific example, but all are children of God, secure in His love. Indeed, all who suffer in tribulation, irrespective of age, are God's beloved children. They are children, because they have humbled themselves or because they have been brought to humility by their experience on earth. But those who lose all in the world gain all in eternity, as they are received into the loving arms of their heavenly Father.

Anthony's legacy for us, in his life and in his death, offers insight into the intractable questions which arise in all human hearts and minds that are plunged into the depths of grief. It is to these that we must turn in the final chapter. For it would surely be Anthony's intention that the understanding of the mystery of life and death he was able to reveal to us in our loss of him, should be available to all who grieve.

Footsteps

Anthony invites us to follow in his footsteps. But in the weakness of our mortality, the very condition that will ultimately impel us on this journey, we stumble at the first step. Our pathway vanishes in the dense fog of confusion filling our exhausted minds. Many members of Anthony's family, in their distress, asked questions that seemed quite impossible to face when we were overwhelmed by the immediate grief of our loss. Now, as the years have passed, it seems a little easier to attempt the task.

The questions raised following the death of a person we love, particularly a child, are fundamental and obdurate. In the welter of our emotion they are obsessive and tormenting. They haunt the mind as spectres that will not be banished. Our minds, attuned to the everyday experience of the humdrum world, do battle with our faith, whether it is weak or strong. However difficult, we have to cling to the reality that our love for the one we have lost is rooted in our hearts; the pain of our broken hearts is the very measure of our love. To follow Anthony we have to perceive the truth with our hearts, just as he saw it. We have to allow ourselves to be possessed by the love of God.

In bereavement, it is scarcely credible that our distraught minds will find any rational answers, as they are torn by the emotion of our loss. We seek consolation as much as understanding. If we are lucky, we may find it in the loving arms of wise friends, who have themselves experienced such sorrow. Only they will know that healing takes much time, that our loss can never be made good in this world and that the individual paths through grief are many. The wisdom they bring us is the first step in the healing of our wounded souls.

Anthony's experience may help us in this healing of the human spirit by pointing us to the right pathway. He certainly hoped so. Anthony knew where he was going; he had no doubt of it and he was confident that we should follow him. True to his nature, there was a little irony in his request; he understood that we should be somewhat confounded by this injunction, but his sense of humour shone through, even here. For Anthony had the advantage of us, he could see the way ahead clearly and he hoped, in the strength of his final revelation, that we should appreciate this. The gift of grace he was given in his experience opened his eyes to the truth. He surely knew that the love his family and friends bore him was the key to the beginning of their understanding.

As our hearts were opened in compassion for the boy we loved, the confusing fog of questions shielding us from healing would start to clear. For Anthony's journey was, and is, a spiritual one, just as the 'answers' to our questions are spiritual. We make progress in the footsteps of our lives when we are close to those we love (and thus to God) in the spirit. If we cannot be present in the spirit to those who are given to us in love, then we are lost. For true love resides in the heart, not in the mind or the emotions.

We have already considered the gift Anthony brought us in our grief in the previous chapter. When death claims a person we love, especially a child, the overwhelming grip of grief is inevitable. For many, this is an unendurable burden; they cannot see how they are ever to live again in their sad loss. As we have seen, grief is the extreme expression of a broken heart. The intensity of grief is in direct proportion to our love for the deceased – the mirror image of that love. To deny grief is to pretend that we never loved; it is the mind's desperate attempt to quell the affliction of the heart.

In the agony of grief, the answers we seek are many and profound. Our basic plea is 'why?' Over and over again, 'why?'; 'how can this happen to me?' We do not know why the pain of grief is so intense. Can grief be avoided in any way? Can we, should we, wish to ease the pain of our suffering in grief? Why do individuals differ so much in the way they grieve? Why do we find it so hard to cope with grief, in ourselves and in others? If grief is a universal human response to the suffering and death of those we love, what is its purpose? Where are we to turn to find healing in our grief? How are we to care for those we love who grieve in anguish?

As we saw in the last chapter, grief that is acceded to and lived through will bring us closer to the one we have lost and it may gradually change our suffering into a vision of certain hope. Grief resisted and struggled with may lead us into bitterness and perhaps even to vengeful anger with God or with whomsoever we blame for our suffering. In the end, such resistance, by closing our hearts, will deny us the healing love of God and subsume grief's bounteous gift of the expression of our momentous love to and for the person we have lost. In effect, such a rebuttal of grief is an attempt to put our own needs first as we try to get over the suffering. The result is to diminish our souls and to reduce our humanity.

Friends and acquaintances, who do not share our grief, though they may wish to help us, will be embarrassed by the raw emotion of our sorrow. They, too, will want us to 'get over it' as quickly as possible; to get 'back to normal'. But that cannot be. We know that we must live through our grief in our own good time and let it change us, as it will. Only our wisest friends will understand this. They will accept our tears and they will comfort us with their quiet and loving presence; for no words can heal a broken heart.

The immediate effect of our grief at Anthony's death was to unite us all, family and friends, in our love for him. His absence was an indescribable pain. As time went by, each person experienced the pain of loss differently. In my own case, the appalling emptiness of loss lasted for some weeks. There was a sickening numbness as the days passed virtually unnoticed. This was replaced quite suddenly by a surprising and overwhelming feeling of love. It was as though I was lifted into the warmth of a loving embrace of an intensity I had never before experienced. I knew that Anthony was with me in this amazing love, as healing of infinite tenderness was applied to my soul. I was able to see Anthony's life as one of the greatest gifts I have ever received. This spiritual experience confirmed for me the immense value of this gentle boy's life. Like so many who knew and loved him, I shall miss him every day, but his brave spirit will never leave my heart. My life has been changed and can never be the same again, because Anthony has touched my soul and the mark he has made will be carried with me forever.

Of course, I cannot speak for others in their loss at Anthony's death. I am sure that there were as many paths through this suffering as there were people. There is no doubt that the ultimate deprivation, a tribulation beyond understanding, was experienced by Gill, Anthony's beloved mother. It is certain that Gill's great love for her only son continues unceasingly, as she now devotes her life to working in Anthony's memory in the bone cancer charity they both started. It was

Anthony's wish that the suffering of the children and young people who are afflicted with this terrible disease should be reduced. Gill's dedicated efforts have been an inspiration to many; not least in the medical profession. Her initiative and boundless hard work have contributed to the founding of a national bone cancer charity, with a rapidly growing international influence. Large amounts of money are being raised and many highly qualified research teams are being funded in an effort to reduce the devastating impact of bone cancer. In time, this will happen. Anthony must be so proud of his mum; their love continues and will never end. It is a love that has resulted in the world being changed for the good of humanity.

Another human emotion evoked by the experience of death is fear. If we pause to think, we marvel at the bravery of each human life, for each life is lived under the ever-present shadow of death. We live under the maxim '*carpe diem*', seize the day, because we know that the very fact of being in the world carries the certainty of not being in it. How are we to escape from the natural fear of death, of those we love and of ourselves? The normal human response to fear is fight or flight. But we cannot run from death and ultimately, we cannot win, however we struggle against it. What is the antidote to fear?

There is nothing more certain than the inevitability of death for each human being and nothing less certain than the moment at which it comes to claim us. In our own society, death is rather a taboo subject. We can only cope with its artificial and its fictional representation in 'murder mysteries' related in book or film. Here, it is formulaic, controllable, removed from our emotions and capable of being switched off at will. The reality of death (particularly of those close to us) is not a topic we are used to dealing with. We do not wish to accept the certainty of death and neither do we wish to consider its implications. For death is a fearsome enemy; unconquerable, capricious, implacable and horrific in its results. Those carried away by its visitation experience no more the beauties and trials of this world and those remaining have the unfathomable loss of their loved ones, the apparent destruction of the very mystery of the life they created together in love. It is all so mysterious, unknowable and meaningless. And we are so afraid of the unknown. Jesus was aware that fear was a basic human instinct; His frequently repeated reassurance to His disciples and to strangers was 'Be not afraid'. In most people, fear cannot be overcome by an act of will. This is testified by the evidence of countless soldiers on the battlefield; neither the toughest training nor the routine of experience will diminish the raw panic of emotion when facing the onslaught of the enemy. Tragically, many people face pain and death in the grip of uncontrollable fear. Others die in peace. There is no rational explanation for this, but we may assume that the strength to face death free of fear may be a gift from God.

This seems to have been the case with Anthony. We have cited the evidence in earlier chapters that he showed no fear of approaching death; we noted his brave example as one of the gifts he bequeaths us. Despite the hurt of his cancer, the aggressiveness of the chemotherapy, the uselessness of his affected leg and his weakness and exhaustion, he showed no fear. He knew what he had to face, but his approach was peaceful, cheerful, balanced and rational. He got through the often uncomfortable routine of each day with a gentle, stolid sobriety. Moreover, unless he was very tired, he had time for a friendly smile and a cheerful word with his many visitors. This, he kept up day after day, knowing that death was rushing towards him with an unstoppable and regular momentum as the days were struck off the calendar. Indeed, as the end approached, he seemed to sense it. He used his awareness as the cue to set his little affairs in order, as witnessed by his gentle farewell talk with Katie and his discussions with his mum about the disposal of his precious models, games, CDs and videos. We are certain that Anthony's peace came from the love in which he lived. At the end, his remarkable revelation confirmed that it was a gift from God, who is love. If we love, we have no need of any fear of death.

If we can set our fear aside, how are we to comprehend death? Why is it a mystery? Why is it inevitable? What is its purpose? What is the reality of death in spiritual terms? The scriptures tell us that our mortality is the price we pay for living in a world where evil deceives human hearts. Anthony's equanimity at his approaching death was remarkable and his final words afford us a glimpse of the transition that death seems to be, certainly in his experience. Our fear of death arises because it is the great unknown, the most profound mystery we have to face. One of the main reasons for the writing of this book is the heartening view of the reality of death that Anthony's evidence gives us. Far from the horrific image created by our temporal culture, Anthony appears to have been rushing into an exciting and beautiful new life; a life in which his whole experience was heightened and joyful. We know that Anthony was an innocent child, but we remember that he was in no way religious. Heaven may be for innocent children, but it does not seem to be reserved for the 'religious' ones only.

What about the rest of us, those who have grown through adulthood with the cares of the world full upon our shoulders? Do we also dare to live in expectation of a transition to a new life after death? Most of us are sinners, but we can live in hope, because of Christ's remarkable promise to us. He came to heal the contrite. He did not come for those who are certain that they are not sinners, but for those who know they are:

> Those who are well have no need of a
> physician, but those who are sick; I have not
> come to call the righteous, but sinners to repentance.
>
> (Luke 5:31–32.)

It is worth remembering Peter's amazing plea to Jesus: 'Begone from me, O Lord, for I am a sinful man'. And Christ's almost breathtaking response: 'Be not afraid'. (Luke 5:8, 10). Peter could not bear to bring his own sinful presence into the balmy aura of his Master's holiness. But it is exactly for us sinners that the Lord brings his balm. He loves us because of His compassion; He sees our desperate need for healing and He understands our weakness. He is the only one who can, at our final hour, bring us to our heavenly Father, so that we may dwell in His light with those we love forever.

The psychologist C. G. Jung believed that the fear of death was intensified when life had lost its deeper meaning, as it has for so many in our time. He also thought that death was a goal towards which we can strive. In other words, life may be seen as a preparation for death. We have seen this truth quite clearly in Anthony's life, as discussed in the previous chapter. Death, it seems, is a paradox, an end and a beginning; a natural transition in our spiritual journey, despite our perfectly understandable apprehension. Even Jesus asked His heavenly Father if the cup of suffering and death might be taken from Him, during His agony of waiting in the Garden of Gethsemane (Matt. 26:38–39).

The problem of suffering is the most powerful argument cited by those who dismiss the reality of a loving God. Either He does not exist or He is a cruel monster: 'As flies to wanton boys are we to the gods, they kill us for their sport' (*King Lear,* Act 4, Scene I). The questions that tore at our hearts as we beheld Anthony in the prison of his hospital bed are familiar to all who endure suffering: Why do the innocent suffer in the world? Why is it that the more we love, the more we suffer – as in grief? How can we equate suffering with God's goodness, as revealed in the life of Jesus? Is tribulation inevitable? Can suffering be avoided? Where can we turn for relief from suffering and for healing from its wounds? There are many more such questions, but the answers we seek are elusive.

We can see that suffering abounds in the world. It comes in many forms, but few lives are untouched by it and for many, life is a journey through a vale of tears. It seems that suffering is an intrinsic part of life, especially of a life lived to the full. Thomas Hardy encapsulates the inexorable nature of tribulation in the final paragraph of his masterpiece *The Mayor of Casterbridge:* 'Her experience had been of a kind to teach her, rightly or wrongly, that the doubtful honour of a brief transit through a sorry world hardly called for effusiveness …. that happiness was but the occasional episode in a general drama of pain'.

Anthony was an innocent child, who was compelled to linger in the valley of the shadow of death. He suffered appallingly and died, for no apparent reason, from a cruel and devastating disease. How are we, who treasured him and loved him, to match this seemingly random tragedy with our faith in a loving God? We might wonder why God (if He is both good and omnipotent) does not intervene; why does He not act to save the world from the evil that appears to infect every aspect of His creation. Jung confirms the view we have of the reality of creation: 'The world is not a garden of God the Father, it is also a place of horror'.

Most children, as they grow and learn, mercifully have a gentle awakening to this 'world of horror'. Little by little, they come to see that people and things are often not quite as nice as the goal to which they themselves have been enjoined to aspire. They learn the ways of the world; their innocence is disabused. Unfortunately, many children are precipitated much more rapidly into the nastiness of the world. Perhaps the world is such a place of uncertain horror, where innocent children may suffer from abuse, accidents, disease and disaster, because human beings, who were created in the image of God, are, in some way, separated from Him. Has our pride and self-confidence caused a division between humans and their Creator? The yearnings of our hearts tell us that we were created to be with God. Instead, we have chosen to love ourselves as we endeavour to manipulate the whole world to our frequently conflicting purposes. As human beings have attempted to become godlike, paradoxically they seem to have lost their own divine inheritance. Do innocent individuals deserve to suffer because humanity in general has lost its way or because there is evil in the world?

The answer must surely be an emphatic 'no'. Anthony was not a child obsessed with himself. He was full of delight at the mystery and wonder of existence. It was his joy to explore God's creation and he was lucky to have a loving family and friends to support and to encourage him. More importantly, as we have seen, his heart was open to the needs of others; he willingly gave and received love from those around him. Anthony did not deserve to suffer, but neither do most people who are hurt so cruelly in the world. Why is this? Why do we have the certainty that the world is, in many senses, an unfitting place for human beings to live in the hope of happiness? Hardy puts it thus: 'But her strong sense that neither she nor any human being deserved less than was given, did not blind her to the fact that there were others receiving less who had deserved much more'. Hardy's concern for the condition of humanity and for the randomness of fate's cruel assaults touches our hearts. If the human heart is so moved by the fate of humanity, what of God's heart?

People do not deserve the suffering they endure. We did not ask to be in a world of suffering and neither did we choose to be weak and broken, so that we are afflicted by our own mistakes and by those of others. The price of love is suffering and the cruelest enigma is that those who love most will almost certainly suffer most. We know from the life of Jesus that God is love. The Son of God healed the suffering and His teaching was sublime. In the Beatitudes (Matt. 5:1–12), we see the divine compassion poured out for the poor, the sick, the bereaved, the gentle, the merciful, the innocent, the peaceful and those who are persecuted. All these, said Jesus, would be rewarded in God's kingdom. How do we resolve the appalling contradiction of a world of horror, where innocents suffer, which has been created by a God of love?

The answer is a mystery, but the wisdom of others may open our eyes and hearts a little, for this is surely a spiritual mystery leading us towards the value and meaning of human life itself which, in its totality, is beyond our comprehension. After his acknowledgement that the world is 'a place of horror', Jung goes on to give us the beginning of a line of consideration, which may lead us towards the light: 'But God himself cannot flourish if man's soul is starved' (i.e. starved of spiritual nourishment). We are brought back full-circle to our alienation from God; we are damaged, because we cut ourselves off from His love and He is damaged because we are incapable of loving Him. Human beings suffer because they live in a damaged creation; for God is existence and if He cannot flourish then neither can the creation He holds in existence. Thus, accidents, disease and natural disasters, the source of so much inexplicable suffering, are not the will of God, but the result of damage to the spiritual reality which is the very foundation and infrastructure of the material world (Jerem. 11:12).

As we beheld Anthony slowly dying before us in the grip of his fearful cancer, we witnessed the destruction by the broken world of the very image of God. For all human beings are made in His image and this divine reflection is never more truly seen than in our suffering children. As our love was torn in our breaking hearts, we were witness to the spiritual sickness brought into the world by the starving of the human soul. God does not want this terrible suffering and neither does He choose those who suffer. But neither does God make mistakes. He gives us freedom to choose (to love Him or not), because the alternative would be to bind His people into slavery. The mystery that God's children suffer in the world under His permissive will is because His love for us cannot be, without our freedom. Love, freedom and suffering are inextricably linked, as in all human relationships.

In Anthony's death, our hopes for him appeared to be dashed. His life held such promise and we believed that so much good would flow from his being in the world. Although the mystery of his death has given us a gloriously fulfilling glimpse of the reality beyond this world, the warmth and love of his physical presence have been taken from us. Can we be compensated for our wounded souls? When we lose our beloved children, do we lose all hope? For our children are the future; our hope rests in them. Indeed, can anyone have any hope in such a fearful world? To whom can we turn for hope? Can we believe that the redemption of the broken creation has begun, because God has entered into the world as a man? In His agony on the Cross, Jesus bears all our grief and also all His Father's grief. God's appalling grief arises from His mighty love for His children, whom He sees suffering in His creation. In one of Jung's most powerful insights (cited by J. Arnold in *Life Conquers Death*), he suggests that the crucifixion is 'God in Christ making reparation to man for a world in which sin and suffering are not only possible, but inevitable'. This is a profound and moving exposition, which opens our eyes to God's overwhelming compassion. In tribulation, He comes to suffer and die in unity with us. In His agony of suffering at what we have endured, God subsumes all our petty mistakes, our weaknesses and our failings. He cries out for our love, our recognition, our compassion, because we are made in His image; we reflect His nature. Surely God's torture, as He endures the world in all its horror, must be the source of our hope? If we can live in God and allow Him to live in us, we shall live in hope as He carries us through our tribulation in the world.

We are certain from Anthony's remarkable witness at the hour of his death, at the summation of all his suffering, that God's almighty love lifted this innocent child into paradise, in complete atonement for all he had so undeservedly endured. We were spared the agony of our heavenly Father's tears, as He beheld the beautiful, loving face of the boy, the son, who held out his arms to caress the Creator of the universe. We are sure that Anthony did not cease to live and to live is to live in hope, to give up hope is to cease to live. Anthony knew we must follow him; in the mystery of his death, he bequeaths us hope and life as he enters into the reality beyond this world.

Thus, in a blessed irony, we who lived through the suffering and death of Anthony were not denied our faith or hope by the depth of this experience. As Brother George observes in the foreword to this book – it was in the mystery of Ant's death that the gift of the fullness of his life was made present to us in the depth of our hearts. That is the Christian paradox he wrote of; our experience of suffering has strengthened our faith and it has brought us closer to Anthony.

There will be many who cannot come to any such resolution of the enigma of suffering. What they endure is simply too overwhelming. Their souls are wounded by the tearing away of all they loved; their hearts devastated by the apparently random and meaningless ravages of fate. Their cruel experience denies their faith or is absolute confirmation of their lack of faith. They will have no understanding of Brother George's 'Christian paradox'.

Questions about faith are frequently uppermost in the minds of the bereaved and this is true, not least, in those who may feel themselves not to be religious in any way; to those who may have a weak faith or none. In our distress, and even anger, we cry, 'How can God let this happen?'

We do not know why He fails to answer our prayers. How can we possibly believe in, or go on believing in, a God who lets innocent children suffer and die? Those who have faith will question its very foundations and those of no faith will be confirmed in their disbelief. But even those who rarely think about faith will be surprised by the force of these considerations at a time of bereavement. For the death of one we love affects not only our physical health, our minds and emotions but, most importantly, our hearts and our spirits. At our time of loss, we find it so difficult to 'cope', because we are brought face-to-face with matters most of us normally do our best to avoid; considerations of the spiritual. It is a time when we have to take account of the very value and meaning of human life. To come to terms with such matters may be very difficult: we may be distressed or feel guilty about our failings in our relationship with the deceased; we may be concerned about the direction and purpose of our own lives. The loss of a person we love brings our deepest feelings to the surface; we find ourselves in uncharted territory. But we may notice in those around us that people who have some faith seem to possess an important key to the comprehension of these difficult questions. They may not have the 'answers' we believe we need, but they are blessed with an inner calmness, a source of strength and consolation for others.

Though Gill, Anthony's mother, does not regard herself as being religious in any way, she has told me that since the death of her beloved son, she does not know how any bereaved parents can possibly cope with their loss in the absence of a belief that there is 'something' beyond death. The importance of faith in the hereafter is, she knows without doubt, essential in allowing her to continue the exhausting challenge of life in this world. It is also the foundation of her abiding loving relationship with Anthony. She is certain of the closeness of his spirit to her. It is a mystery, but their love endures and it is the basis of the strength that sustains Gill in her loss.

Anthony was not a regular churchgoer, and neither did he spend much time beyond scripture lessons engrossed in the pages of the Bible. He was not 'religious' in the conventional sense. His faith was that of an innocent child; his selfless love in his suffering, the prevenient grace of eternal life. We, who love him, are transformed by Anthony's gift to us and as we follow him, we are guided into the reality beyond this world. Those with faith have found it strengthened by the mystery of Anthony's life and death. He has brought us closer to the inscrutable God of compassion and love, who has lifted him into eternity. It seems likely, as Anthony endured his suffering, that his nearness to God increased; the strength of God's love calling to him was surely irresistible. Anthony had no doubts about the direction in which he was heading. I am sure that during his long illness he was drawn nearer to God in the bond of suffering and love. At his final hour, his words reveal that he came into the presence of perfect love. If he knew God, as his experience suggests, then his faith was made perfect also, for to know God is to have absolute faith.

Why do some people have faith in God and others do not? This question brings us to the relationship between our minds and our hearts. Anthony certainly used his mind. He was keen on all the sciences and he did well in them at school. He was particularly good at the practical application of physics, especially electronics. Even while ill in bed, he was constructing a somewhat complex robot using skills of mind and delicacy of hand. Unfortunately, though his robot reached the stage of perambulating around his bed under radio control from Ant, he did not have time to finish it. I still have his robot, as a treasured reminder of Anthony, but I do not think I shall ever complete it – though one day Anthony is sure to ask me why I failed to do so! But Anthony's heart was also open and put to good use. We have witnessed his numerous acts of kindness, in particular his concern for his family and his care for his school friends, as related in the first chapter. Anthony's spiritual awareness at the end of his life is clinching evidence of the fullness of his experience; his openness to God. This is the necessary prerequisite to faith, for faith is a gift from God.

When we are given this wonderful gift, it opens our eyes to see the truth of God in the light of our faith. St Augustine taught that it is not by understanding that we come to faith, but by faith that we come to understanding. We understand that we do not have to prove God's existence; for He does not have existence, He is existence. True faith is based on the experience that God gives us and we can only experience His love when our hearts are open; that is when we are present to Him in the spirit. The gift of faith gives us a new vision of reality as heart and mind together open the eyes of understanding. This is the truth that is given to children and which is denied to many wise men. God's children, like Katie and Anthony, see the world, and especially the people in it, in the light of love. It is by God's grace that we have the gift of faith; it is the manna, which nourishes our hearts – our souls no longer starve. In effect, faith is the gift of God's presence in our hearts. As Jung tells us: 'In religious matters we cannot understand a thing until we have experienced it inwardly'. But the gift of faith carries a responsibility. There is a price to be paid for accepting God's love. If Christ enters our hearts, we live with Him and we suffer with Him. The grace of faith is the gift of the Cross. When we accept the Lord's gift of faith, He is choosing us as He chose His disciples. As with the twelve He chose in Galilee, we cannot expect our lives to be easy or unchanged. Far from damaging our faith, the mystery of Anthony's death has given us a direct internal experience of God. Our love of Anthony has led us with him into the reality of eternal love. Anthony's story offers us the rare opportunity to align faith with experience; perhaps the most earnest need of humankind as we live through the enigma of our mortal lives in a secular and materialistic world.

In the end, the ultimate answer to our loss is surrender, to abandon ourselves to love. For the love of the one we mourn is a measure of our humanity, a reflection of the God in whose image we are all made. Anthony was one of countless innocent children who suffer and die in our disordered world. As he approached the end of his mortal life, enfolded in his mother's arms, his final words convince us in our faith that the Lord came to this gentle boy, taking away his pain and filling him with joy and peace. In the world, Anthony had lived in love and for love. In his final moments, love came for him and, as his words reveal, captivated him in wonder and delight.

Epilogue

Anthony has caused us to rethink our own life-journeys, because we are transformed by his experience and because we know that one day, we shall have to follow him through the gateway of death. In the last chapter we have examined the distressing impact of bereavement and the contribution of Anthony's experience to our response. Here, we return to the essence of Anthony's own witness, to the brave boy whose terrible suffering and enigmatic vision at the hour of his death has brought about our awakening from the slumber of our lives. The glimpses Anthony has given us of the mysteries beyond this world have been a sure sign of the need for the reordering of our priorities in the brief transit of our mortal lives. The conclusions we draw from this little lad's experiences bring us no less than face-to-face with the most profound questions of life and death, with the meaning of our existence and with the nature of our relationship with the supernatural world, which exists beyond and above us.

Anthony's story illustrates the importance of the spirituality of those approaching death and especially of terminally ill children. There is a growing awareness of the significance of the spiritual dimension in the palliative care of children. Each child's spiritual experience as he or she approaches death is surely unique. Those who love and care for dying children know that the world alone can provide no 'answers' for the children, for ourselves or for others. Death is, and will remain, a mystery. But our faith allows us to place our hope in the promise of the risen Christ.

Above all, what Anthony's life and death have given us is an understanding of the eternal presence of God in His own beloved Son. We know it is the closeness of Jesus which alone can bring us peace and truth in life and death. As we consider the stages of Anthony's journey, we believe that the Lord was with him at each step, holding him in love and guiding him into his new life. St Bernard of Clairvaux saw the presence of Christ as being like a road leading from His suffering and death to His final coming in glory at the end of time. As did Anthony, we travel the same road in hope, from the suffering flesh to the glory of resurrection.

We believe that the Lord's friendship guided Anthony from first to last, on his journey through tribulation to his heavenly home. The nearness of Jesus shines through the gentleness and humour of the boy's early life. His love came in the consoling appearance of the 'angel' seen by Ant as he lay in his bed of suffering. Anthony's request to 'follow me' at his funeral reflects Christ's own invitation as He guides us to paradise.

At Anthony's final hour, his remarkable vision and his words of joy as he played with his 'superheroes' suggests the compassionate attention of the Son of God as the boy prepares to take the momentous concluding steps in his journey. It seems, from Ant's words, that God, in His omniscient love, plumbs the depths of the souls of His beloved children as they come to Him, granting them, in His boundless generosity, all they could ever wish for. St Bernard tells us that the Lord comes to be with us 'in the spirit and in power'. If this is so, we may begin to understand how the boy's spirit was lifted from his body into the freedom that is the will of God. We glimpse the omnipotence of God, who uses His mighty power to rescue His beloved children from their tribulation. He removes them from the constraints of time and space as He brings them to live in His light.

We see also, in Anthony's vision, the importance to our Lord of loving relationships. The 'lovely lady', who came to Ant and who was so full of kindness, was in her companionship and love the expression of God's unbelievable gentleness in His relationship with us. God is the Lord of relationships; He lives in and with our relationships at all times; He is omnipresent. He exists in the mystery of the Trinity as an everlasting relationship of love.

As we were close to Anthony at his bedside, in our love for him we brought him the only comfort we could give and all he needed in earthly terms. We were full of humility as we responded to the needs of the boy we loved, who lay at heaven's gate. We knew we were preparing him, simply by our presence, to return into the tender arms of his heavenly Father, the One who had created him. No doubt he was gently taken to those welcoming arms by the lovely lady, who continued his mother's loving warmth as he passed beyond our reach.

We know that in our minds, we cannot answer satisfactorily all those difficult questions about the suffering and loss of those we love. The 'answers' are to be found in our hearts. In our prayer, we place those we love in God's care. We know that His closeness is the only answer to all our needs and the needs of those we love. As human beings decline into the utter powerlessness of death, we see the paradox of Christ's immense power. He who was killed by the brutal, physical power of the world and offered no resistance as He was raised on the Cross was undefeated; He rose again:

> And I, when I am lifted up from the earth,
> will draw all men to myself.
>
> (John 12:32.)

His raising on the Cross and His raising into new life are the inseparable sources of the salvation offered by Jesus to all human beings. It is His presence in the power of the resurrection that we rely upon to be lifted into eternity with Him. This gift of Christ is the transcendence of man to reach God. We have seen it happen as our beloved children, like Anthony, are received into the new life that our Lord has won for them at the end of their brief sojourn on this earth. We grieve for the suffering they have endured and for our loss, but we can be certain that we are with them in love, as they live in perpetual delight with the Lord of the universe.

At the last, with Anthony, we shall come into the presence of the One who made the heavens and the earth. The presence of God is our eternal destiny. We are able to come into His presence, who is spirit, when we ourselves are present in the spirit. To be so we open our hearts to Him in love as we ask for His mercy. His love brings us all our needs and all our gifts in life. It is His gift of faith that brings us close to Him; His gift of prayer which strengthens our faith; His gift of His Word which speaks the truth to us; His gift of the Church and its sacraments that allows us to touch Him; and, in the end, His gift of redemption that brings us into His everlasting presence. In life and death, all is grace.

In Anthony's brave journey, what we have seen is the transforming power of God's touch. Anthony has witnessed to his own transcendence at the hour of his death. As with every true witness, God has spoken to us, offering His redeeming message of love and hope. We are changed by this gift of grace and we know that our Lord's invitation, 'Follow Me', will be our guide and our salvation. In His presence, He will bring us to His Father's house, where we shall abide in love, reunited in joy with our beloved Anthony and with all those we have lost in the world:

> In the beginning was the Word,
> and the Word was with God,
> and the Word was God.
> He was in the beginning with God;
> all things were made through him,
> and without him was not anything made that was made.
> In him was life, and the life was the light of men.
> The light shines in the darkness,
> and the darkness has not overcome it.
>
> (John 1:1–5.)

Postscript – Bone Cancer

Introduction

Anthony died of osteosarcoma. This is one of the two most common forms of primary bone cancer, the other being Ewing's sarcoma. The primary bone cancers are cancers that arise within bone cells, rather than spreading from other sites.

Types and Numbers Affected

Both of these cancers affect bones, but osteosarcoma arises from malfunctioning bone-producing cells (osteoblasts), whereas Ewing's sarcoma arises from other bone cells. In Britain, there has been no real change for many years in the numbers affected by these cancers. For example, while bone cancer numbers remain static, the number of people affected by brain tumours is increasing. In the UK, there are between 150 and 200 new cases of osteosarcoma a year and about eighty cases of Ewing's sarcoma. Both of these cancers almost always occur in children and young people. If we include the more unusual types of bone cancer, we arrive at an annual total of about 400 newly diagnosed cases of primary bone cancer per year in the UK.

Osteosarcoma occurs most frequently at puberty, usually at the ends of the limb bones, which are growing rapidly at this time. The ends of the femur (the upper leg bone), particularly the lower end near the knee, grow most rapidly and are especially prone to developing osteosarcoma tumours. (Anthony's tumour was at this site.) The arm bones can also be affected, other bones more rarely. Ewing's sarcoma (named after the doctor who first described it) also seems to be related in some way to periods of rapid bone growth. The most common sites for it are bones of the pelvis, thigh, lower leg, upper arms and ribs.

Because they are cancers of rapidly growing bone, these tumours are found most commonly in children and young adults. Osteosarcoma has a peak occurrence between the ages of 15 and 20 years, though it can occur in young children and in older adults; Ewing's sarcoma has a wider age range, typically between 10 and 20 years old. It can also arise in very young children and in older adults.

Fig.1. Approximate Age Distribution of Primary Bone Cancers

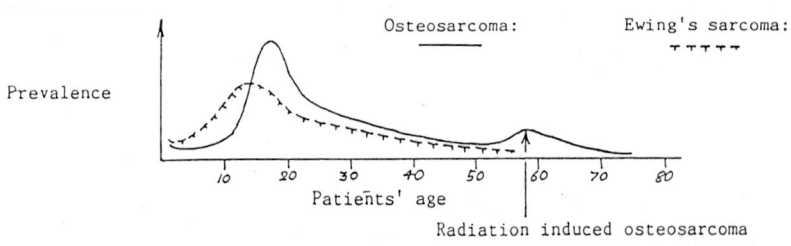

The second peak in the curve for osteosarcoma, at around the age of 60, is believed to be the result of radiation induction, possibly arising from earlier treatment.

Symptoms and Diagnosis

Because bone cancers are comparatively rare, GPs frequently fail to recognise them. It usually takes a long time from first symptoms to diagnosis. The symptoms of both of these cancers are increasing pain and local swelling at the site of the tumour. Osteosarcoma is more painful and this comes on more quickly than Ewing's sarcoma. From symptoms to diagnosis can take from six weeks to six months for osteosarcoma and from three to nine months for Ewing's sarcoma. Almost all families do make several approaches to the medical services before correct diagnosis. This is well known to the professionals, but what to do about it is a difficult question. There is a clear need for research on this issue, as delay in diagnosis may allow metastasis, the spreading of cancerous cells to other parts of the body, considerably reducing the chances of survival.

Treatment, Outcomes and Survival

In the late 1960s and the early 1970s, before effective chemotherapy, if the patients had no metastasis, the only option was amputation of the affected limb. Despite this, about 90 per cent of patients relapsed with lung sarcoma (secondary tumours in the chest) within a year. Survival with amputation alone was about 10 to 15 per cent. Chemotherapy was introduced in the 1970s and between 1975 and 1981, it was tried after amputation. Following collaboration between American and European specialists, it was found that if initial chemotherapy was given to shrink the tumour, it was much easier to remove it, allowing the possibility of replacing the affected bone with a prosthesis. This method gained in favour because it avoided the need for amputation, which was extremely distressing for patients and their families. In the USA in the 1980s, it was discovered that the initial chemotherapy did not work in about 25 per cent of patients. Because their tumours did not shrink, these patients had to undergo amputation. Since then, chemotherapy has improved, so that amputation can be avoided in most cases.

In Germany and the USA, survival rates are about 4 to 5 per cent better than in the UK, though we don't know the reason for this. Obviously, there is a need for research on variations in survival rates. Patients with identified metastasis have a 42 per cent death rate within a year in Britain, compared to 32 per cent in Germany. Again, we do not know why. With modern treatments, up to 70 per cent of non-metastasised patients may survive and up to 30 per cent of metastasised patients. Unfortunately, about 20 per cent of young people diagnosed with osteosarcoma already have advanced-stage metastasis, usually spreading to the lungs. Generally, the current survival rate in the UK for osteosarcoma is 55 per cent at five years from diagnosis and for Ewing's sarcoma about 60 per cent at five years.

Fig 2. Survival Rate for Bone Cancers

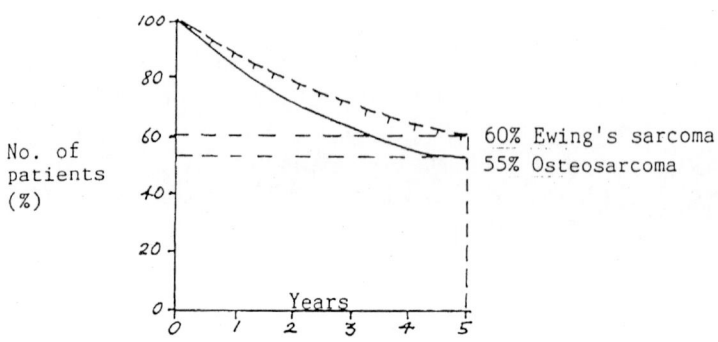

60% Ewing's sarcoma
55% Osteosarcoma

Perhaps the Germans and Americans are better organised than Britain or perhaps they are better at diagnosis. The average size of sarcoma tumours diagnosed in the UK is 10 cm, which is far too large. So we need to know the answers to the questions about why we are performing less well than other countries. We need to lift awareness in the public and in GPs. Large tumours presented late may be the reason for our poor performance in the UK. Early presentation and diagnosis is vital. In Italy, for example, you would get an X ray immediately that there was any suspicion, without any delay.

Present chemotherapy treatments are intensive, they can be disabling and they have no guarantee of success. In the UK, primary bone cancers do not attract extensive research funding from the NHS or national cancer charities. There is little research into the causes of primary bone cancers or into developing new treatments. When a cancer is comparatively rare, the drug companies do not have the incentive of a large potential market to encourage expensive research and development.

Research and Possible Causes

In Britain, there are two major centres for osteosarcoma research, at Stanmore and Birmingham. Research into Ewing's sarcoma is done at Leeds. There are many practical and political issues affecting research and its funding.

Little is known of the causes of bone cancers, but it is probable that in many cases, there are multiple causes, including predetermined genetic propensity. There seems to be a clear genetic link in about 10 per cent of osteosarcoma cases. There are certain cancer syndromes associated with osteosarcoma, e.g. retinoblastoma (eye cancer). About 40 per cent of patients with this condition have a genetic abnormality, which predisposes them to osteosarcoma. They have this abnormality in all of their cells, including their sex cells, so they can pass it on and they have a high risk of getting secondary cancers. It is possible that about 5 per cent of osteosarcoma cases arise from this particular genetic abnormality. Some 90 per cent of osteosarcomas arise sporadically and we do not know why. With around 400 cases a year in the UK, primary bone tumours are not commonplace cancers. This is fortunate for young people, but it emphasises the effort we must put into raising the profile of this badly diagnosed and highly dangerous disease which, because it targets the young, has particularly devastating effects on the families involved. There is an urgent need for much research.

Rob Grimer, a surgeon from Birmingham specialising in bone cancers, has founded the British Sarcoma Group (See www.bsgconference.org.uk or www.sarcoma-uk.org). This is aimed at all the professionals involved, in order to raise the profile of primary bone cancers. Rob Grimer believes that for the last thirty years, we have been using a 'sledgehammer' treatment in the form of chemotherapy. The advantage of intensive chemotherapy is that it is so powerful that it can destroy all the pathways available for the tumour to grow and spread. Its tremendous disadvantage is its extremely debilitating effect on the patient, who is effectively being poisoned, in the hope that the tumour will die before the patient succumbs to the side effects of the drug. New biological agents are just starting to be developed which may eventually allow designer drugs, targeted at specific tumours. As we still rely on very crude treatments, there is a pressing need for more detailed research and development, which could help to move us towards such targeted agents. Although cancer cells are very effective at getting around targeted drugs, the specific anti-cancer drug would be the ideal for effective treatment, with minimum side effects for the patient. This is the goal for the future.

What can be done?Possible areas for research

As we ask questions about the primary bone cancers, groups of issues are raised, which lead on to various research approaches:

QUESTIONS	ISSUES RAISED
a) Why and where?	Epidemiological issues.
b) How many?	Epidemiological issues.
c) Survival?	Epidemiological issues.
d) Improving survival.	Clinical studies and laboratory research.
e) Improving treatment.	Clinical studies & lab research + health services research.
f) Improving diagnosis.	Clinical studies & lab research + health services research.
g) Understanding the disease	New treatments and translational research.
h) Providing information to GPs & public.	Health services and charities.
i) Support for patients & families.	Health services and charities.
j) Fundraising.	Charities.
k) Quality of care.	Health services.

- Epidemiological issues: these are concerned with the study of the patterns of disease, e.g. why does it happen, when, where and how? How many survive? What is the pattern of distribution? Are there any clusters? This is a science involving detailed and complex research. It is linked to accurate registry, i.e. it depends upon the register of cases that have been recorded. The register must be comprehensive and correct. It should record all the relevant data: genetic factors, trauma, prenatal exposure to radiation, other exposures, lifestyle of child and family, medical history of child and family, etc.

- Clinical studies and laboratory research: clinical studies and trials concern the testing of new treatments as they become available. The British are quite good at this, but pharmacological companies are not too keen on funding studies into rare cancers such as osteosarcoma. It can take many years to do a worthwhile clinical trial. Laboratory research allows us to understand the disease, e.g. at Leeds, Ian Lewis and his team are looking at how cancers grow by stimulating blood vessel growth. This is called angiogenesis and it is important in cancers in general.

- New treatments and translational research: the better we understand the disease the more we can help new treatments to be developed. Translational research is basic lab research which aims to relate clinical issues to the new research findings. In this way, the lab research translates into new and potentially useful treatments the clinicians can use.

- The National Health Service: we need to consider how we can make the health service work more efficiently. All the people working in the service need to be better informed. GPs need the correct, up-to-date information. The public need to be given all the relevant information. In the UK, it sometimes seems as though the health service works as a sort of financial gatekeeper, screening out expensive, rare diseases such as the primary bone cancers. If primary care was organised differently, we might see a greatly improved outcome. In Germany and France there is a totally different approach, putting the patients first. In the UK, the health service is put first, so that it holds all the cards and is very much in control. The patients and the professionals feel they are in the grip of the organisation, which is primarily concerned with finance. It is as though the priority is to protect the health service from unnecessary investigation.

- Charities: formerly, there was not a national bone cancer charity, but recently this has changed, with the founding of the Bone Cancer Research Trust (see below). Basically, all medical charities are concerned with four interrelated activities, though they may decide to concentrate on one or more of these:

Fig 3. Basic Charity Activities

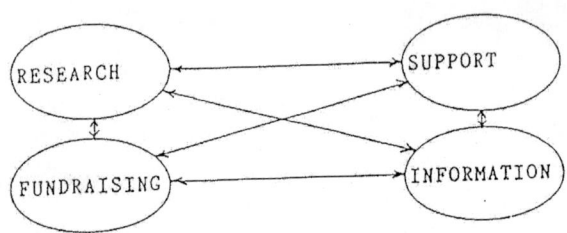

The Anthony Pilcher Bone Cancer Trust (APBCT)

The Anthony Pilcher Bone Cancer Trust (APBCT)

21 Victoria Avenue

Peacehaven

East Sussex

BNIO 8LX

Tel: 01273808874

Fax: 02380 988435

Email: gill@apbonecancertrust.org.uk

Website: www.apbonecancertrust.org.uk

Registered Charity No.: 1099337

The precursor to this charity was instituted by Anthony in April 2001, shortly after he had been diagnosed with osteosarcoma. When the details of his treatment had been explained to him, he discussed with his mum the possibility of establishing a fund, with the hope of reducing the suffering and improving the likely outcome for children who would be similarly diagnosed in future. His first act was to seek sponsorship, as he intended to have his head shaved to pre-empt the hair loss that would be the inevitable result of the chemotherapy; the whole event to be recorded in photographs! I still have a copy of the sponsor form signed by Anthony, with his own touching explanation at the head of the sheet:

> 'I am Tony, I am 14 years old and I live in Peacehaven in Sussex. About 3 weeks ago, a tumour was found in my leg. Shortly after, the tumour was confirmed as malignant. I now know that I will have a six-month course of chemotherapy and an operation to remove the tumour. I am hoping that you will consider sponsoring me to have my hair shaved off during my treatment. All the money raised will be going to cancer research. Thanking you very much for your help.'

Tony Pilcher

Because of Anthony's school nickname 'Fish', the charity was first known as 'Fish Aid'. It evolved from numerous concerts, usually held at Ant's school and arranged by his schoolmate Lewis. The school has continued in its faithful support of Fish Aid including, in recent years, sponsored walks, which have made a fine contribution to the charity's funds.

The first steps were taken to establish a formal charity in a provisional meeting held at Lewes Old Grammar School on 11 March 2003. Anthony's mum Gill worked hard at setting up and registering the new charity. The first trustee meeting of the Anthony Pilcher Bone Cancer Trust was held at LOGS on 9 March 2004. The trust has become a well-supported local charity and it continues to be hosted by LOGS for regular trustee meetings.

The aims of the charity are:

- to raise awareness of this devastating cancer of children and young people;

- to do all that is possible to improve diagnosis and thus to increase the chances of survival;

- to finance research into the causes and treatment of bone cancer;

- to provide support and information for families of young people suffering from primary bone cancer.

Anthony's cancer trust is his most practical legacy to all the young people who are suffering and who will come to suffer from this terrible cancer. Many people have given and continue to give generously in his memory and for the relief of those who suffer as he did. But there is still much work to be done in understanding this cancer and in improving the methods of treatment available.

The APBCT sees itself as a local activity, raising funds in the area of Sussex which was Anthony's home territory. Through Gill's tireless efforts, Anthony's charity has now become one of the founding and satellite members of the new national charity, The Bone Cancer Research Trust (see below). All funds raised by the APBCT are donated to the national charity in Anthony's memory, along with those of several other satellite charities, similarly run by bereaved parents working in local areas.

The Bone Cancer Research Trust (BCRT)

Bone Cancer Research Trust (BCRT)
Fundraising & Administrative Office
Gledhow Mount Mansion
Roxholme Grove
Leeds
LS7 4JJ
Tel: 0113 262 1852
Email: info@bonecancerresearch.org.uk
Website: www.bonecancerresearch.org.uk
Registered Charity No.: 1113276

This new and much-needed national bone cancer charity was initiated by a telephone call from Gill Pilcher (Anthony's mum) to Dr (now Professor) Ian Lewis at St James's University Hospital, Leeds. Professor Lewis is a specialist consultant in bone cancers and Gill rang him to clarify her own understanding of these sarcomas, so that she could be of more help to parents who were contacting the APBCT. Professor Lewis thought that some serious research into these cancers needed initiating and moving ahead with some real pressure. So when Gill rang him, he saw her call as the hoped-for start of some new developments. It seems that Gill's call was very timely. Her initiative was the spark that was to lead to a large, joint enterprise. Ros and Mike Francis from York, parents of Guy, who had been treated by Dr Lewis, were also keen to be involved. On 25 September 2004, Dr Lewis chaired an initial meeting at St James's Hospital and from this, the national charity has grown. Many interested 'satellite' charities, families, former patients, professionals and friends have been involved in the establishment of the new charity and several have become trustees. The BCRT sets out its agenda under a number of headings:

Why is a research trust needed?

Current treatments are intensive, they can be disabling and they have no guarantee of success. There is little research into the causes and treatment of primary bone cancer or into developing new treatments.

What is the Bone Cancer Research Trust?

The trust was formed in 2005 as an alliance of a number of established local charities and groups of families and friends of primary bone cancer patients throughout Britain and Ireland. They share a common goal – to promote research into the causes and treatment of primary bone cancer and, in particular, osteosarcoma and Ewing's sarcoma. The trust has now widened its membership to include bone cancer patients, medical practitioners and anyone interested in supporting research into these disabling and life-threatening diseases. The trust is also hoping to provide information and support and, in the longer term, counselling services for those suffering from primary bone cancer and their families.

What happens to the funds raised?

The trustees' main aim is to raise and distribute funds to research projects or programmes which address the causes, behaviour or treatment of primary bone cancers. Funds will only be distributed following the advice of the Scientific Advisory Panel. This group is made up of distinguished medical practitioners and scientists, who support the aims and purposes of the trust and who have many years' experience in treating or researching into the treatment of cancer.

Who are the founding members?

Adam Dealey Foundation for Ewing's Sarcoma. (Hemel Hempstead, diagnosed age 9.)

Anthony Pilcher Bone Cancer Trust. (Brighton, diagnosed age 14.)

Christopher Hardman Osteosarcoma Research Fund. (Wirral, diagnosed age 13.)

Guy Francis Bone Cancer Research Fund. (York, diagnosed age 17.)

Family and Friends of Krystle Smith. (Arklow, Ireland, diagnosed age 17.)

Family and Friends of Emma Callar. (Helston, Cornwall, diagnosed age 17.)

Family and Friends of Stephanie McCartney. (Keighley, diagnosed age 13.)

Family and Friends of Joe Thompson. (Kettering, diagnosed age 11.)

Family and Friends of Jennifer Carvell. (Liverpool, diagnosed age 13.)

Who is on the Scientific Advisory Panel?

The panel evaluates submissions for research funding, before making recommendations to the Board of Trustees. The panel includes:

Professor Ian Lewis, MB ChB FRCP FRCPCH. Consultant Paediatric and Adolescent Oncologist, St James's University Hospital, Leeds. Past Chair, Medical Research Council (Bone Sarcoma Committee) and United Kingdom Children's Study Group (Bone Sarcoma Group). Mr Robert Grimer MB BS FRCS (Eng) FRCS (Edin) Orth. Consultant Orthopaedic Surgeon, Royal Orthopaedic Hospital, Birmingham. Chair, Sarcoma Group, National Cancer Research Institute Network. Past President, British Orthopaedic Oncology Society. Dr Jeremy Whelan MD MB BS FRCP. Consultant Medical Oncologist and Clinical Director for Cancer Services, Meyerstein Institute of Oncology, University College Hospital, London. Current Chair, NCRI and CCLG, Bone Sarcoma Groups.

Who are the Trustees?

The trustees are drawn from medical practitioners, bone cancer patients and families and friends of those who have, or have had, primary bone cancer:

Nicholas Bones (former bone cancer patient)

John Dealey (parent)

Michael Francis (parent)

Fiona Foley (parent)

Robert Grimer FRCS (consultant orthopaedic surgeon)

Patrick Hardman (parent)

Sally Hurst (former bone cancer patient)

Professor Ian Lewis FRCP (consultant paediatric & adolescent oncologist)

Gill Pilcher (parent)

Patricia Smith (parent)

Links to other cancer organisations:

The Children's Cancer and Leukaemia Group (CCLG)
National Alliance of Childhood Cancer Parent Organisations (NACCPO)
National Cancer Research Institute Network (Sarcoma Group)
Candlelighters, Yorkshire.
Sarcoma UK
Teenagers and Young Adults with Cancer

How you can help: by joining or supporting the trust, you will be helping to raise awareness of the 400 new cases of primary bone cancer in children and young people which occur every year. If you can help to raise funds you will be contributing to the much-needed research campaign. If you would like to contribute to funds, your donation would be gratefully received and will help to further the vital but expensive research programme now under way. Please contact the address mentioned earlier.

Any Royalties arising from the sale of this book will be donated directly to the Anthony Pilcher Bone Cancer Trust.

BONE CANCER
RESEARCH TRUST©
Devoted to promoting research into
the causes and treatment of
Primary Bone Cancer,
and in particular of
Osteosarcoma and Ewing's Sarcoma

Bibliography

Arnold, John. *Life Conquers Death*. Grand Rapids: Zondervan, 2007

Bolt, Robert. *A Man for All Seasons*. Oxford: Heinemann Educational, 1970.

Br. Francis. *Oxford Textbook of Palliative Care for Children*. (Ed. Goldman, Hain and Liben.) Oxford University Press, 2006. Ref: Chapter 6, *The Spiritual Life*.

Foakes, R. A. (Editor) *King Lear*. The Arden Shakespeare, London: Thomson Learning, 1997.

Harding, D. E. *Religions of The World*. London: Heinemann Educational Books Ltd., 1966.

Hardy, Thomas. *The Mayor of Casterbridge*. London: Penguin Popular Classics, 1994.

Holy Bible, Revised Standard Version. The British & Foreign Bible Society, 1967

Jerusalem Bible. Darton, Longman & Todd Ltd. and Doubleday, 1966

Jung, C. G. *Psychological Reflections*. London: Routledge & Kegan Paul, 1971.

Scott Peck, M, *The Road Less Travelled*. London: Arrow Press, 1990.

St Bernard of Clairvaux. *Fifth Sermon on Advent*. Office of Readings for Wednesday, Week 1 of Advent.

Walsh, William Thomas. *Our Lady of Fatima*. New York: Image Books, Doubleday & Co, 1954. (Walsh gives by far the best account of the events at Fatima and I have drawn my brief summaries of 'the angel' and of 'Our Lady' from his work.)

Wells, Samuel. *Power and Passion*. Grand Rapids: Zondervan, 2007.

Music:

Uncle Kracker. *Follow Me*. 757-83279-2. WEA International Inc., 2000